THE OFFICIAL BRITISH ARMY FITNESS GUIDE

Sam Murphy

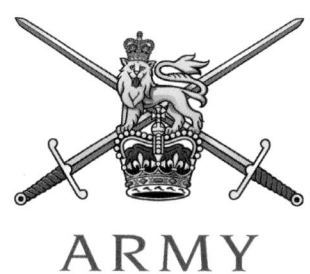

ARMY

First published by Guardian News and Media 2008
This edition published by Guardian Books 2009
Guardian Books is an imprint of Guardian News and Media, 119 Farringdon
Road, London EC1R 3ER
guardianbooks.co.uk

A CIP catalaogue for this book is available from the British Library.

ISBN: 978-0-85265-118-6

Cover and design concept: Gavin Brammall
Edited, designed and set by Essential Works
Photographs by Andy Hall and Eddie Macdonald

Printed and bound in Italy by L.E.G.O. S.p.A.

With thanks to UK Gear and Powerbag for providing clothing and
equipment in support of this book.

Thanks to the staff of Headquarters Army Physical Training Corps and the staff and
students of the Army School of Physical Training, Aldershot for their contributions to
this book; with particular thanks to Martin ColClough, Al Lucas and Al Billings.

Contents

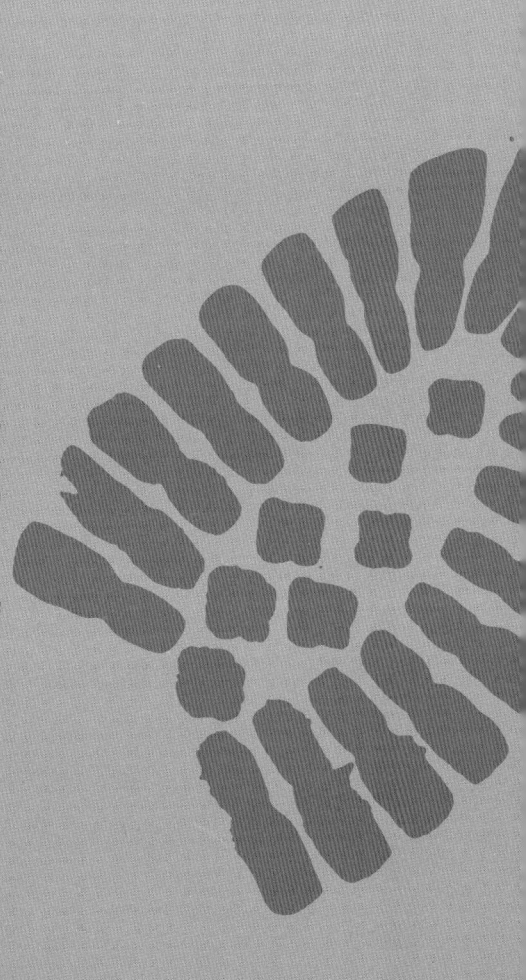

Part One: The Basics 14

Aerobic fitness 16
Strength 34
Stretching and flexibility 78
Warming up and cooling down 94

Part Two: The Programmes 110

Assessing your fitness level 112
Which programme is right for you? 118
Exercise Programme Level One 124
Exercise Programme Level Two 132
Exercise Programme Level Three 140

Part Three: The Practicalities 148

Staying healthy 150
Nutrition and performance 156
Clothing, footwear and equipment 164
Staying motivated 170

Glossary 174

Introduction

Welcome to the *Official British Army Fitness Guide*. If you are looking for a simple, effective way to get fitter, healthier and stronger, you've come to the right place.

The British Army has long been a pioneer in developing fitness plans for its soldiers. More than 150 years ago, following the Crimean War, it set about building the first "Army Gymnastic Staff". The benefits of the training it offered - which included boxing, fencing, gymnastics and general physical activity - were soon apparent, and by 1862 it was decided that there should be a gym in every garrison, with its own officer and instructional staff. The official *Manual of Physical Training* for the Army was first published in 1908.

Of course, things have moved on since then, but today's Physical Training Instructors (PTIs), while keeping well abreast of the latest sport science developments, have stayed true to the fundamentals of exercise proven to be effective through the ages.

The fitness programmes in this book go right back to basics because, in the Army's experience, that's what works. Many exercise regimes in the civilian world are too complicated, too inflexible or require too much equipment. Others take too long, or promise benefits that they simply cannot deliver.

But do not think that a straightforward, no-frills approach to getting fit is the easy option. Based on the actual activities used by the Army Physical Training Corps, these programmes have been developed and modified to suit everyone, from the beginner to the weekend warrior looking to take their fitness to the next level.

Nor does back to basics mean mundane or boring. The Army Physical Training Corps evaluates new exercise methods and equipment, introducing the best of what it finds into its training to keep military personnel on their toes and help them stay motivated. You can be sure that if these programmes work for the Army, they can work for you, too.

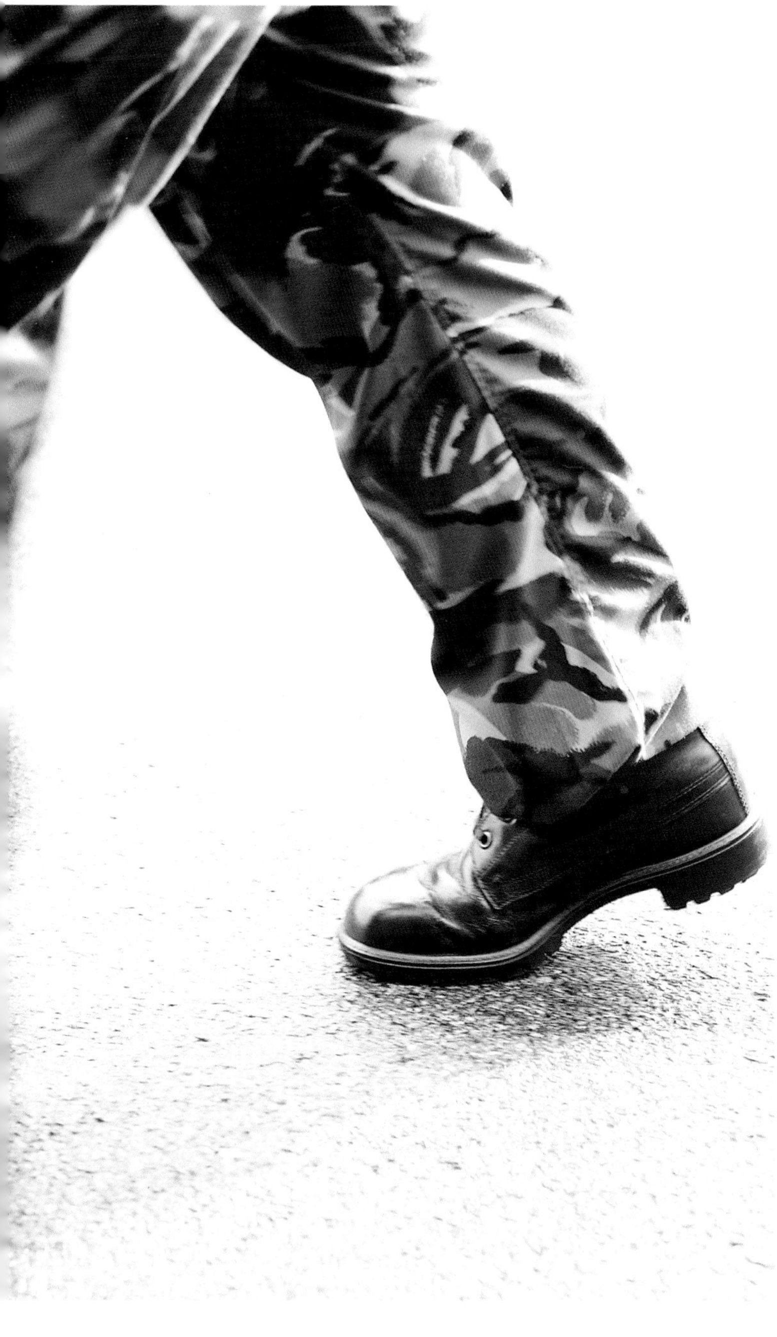

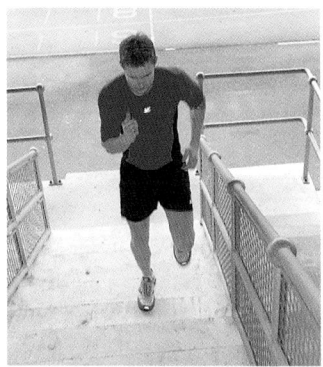

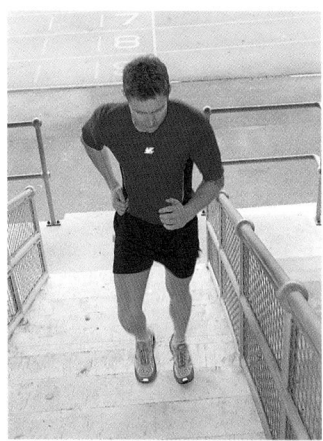

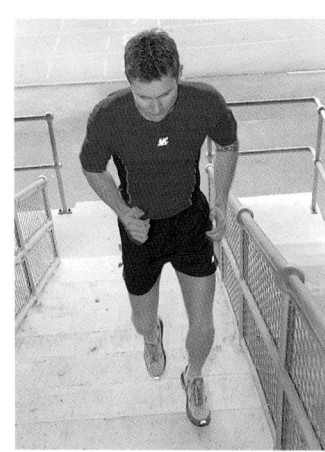

Why the British Army Fitness Guide works

- It is easy to follow and requires little or no equipment.
- It is balanced, so that it works on all aspects of fitness.
- It is suitable for all, because there are different levels of challenge to choose from.
- It is convenient, so can easily be worked into your daily routine.
- It is progressive, ensuring you continue to make improvements.
- It is varied, so you will stay interested and motivated.

How to use this book

The Official British Army Fitness Guide is divided into three parts - The Basics, The Programmes and The Practicalities.

Part One introduces you to the three main components of fitness – aerobic fitness (stamina), strength and flexibility. You will find out what benefits each of these aspects of fitness brings, both in terms of physical performance and improvements to daily life and health. Spend some time understanding correct technique and training methods and, if you are new to that type of exercise, put it all into practice using the four-week "start-up" programmes for each component.

In Part Two, you will move on to the official Army Fitness Programmes. Refer back to the Strength section (pp.34-77) for illustrated descriptions of all the exercises that feature in the programmes. Each of the three 12-week programmes contains workouts designed for a different level of physical fitness - so you will find something for you, whatever your starting point, and the opportunity to move from one programme to the next as your fitness improves. If you reach the end of the most advanced programme your fitness will be comparable to that of a trained soldier.

Part Three looks at the practicalities of safe, effective and successful exercise. It includes advice on how to exercise without getting injured and how to fuel your physical efforts with the right nutrition and hydration strategies. At the end of the book you will find a guide to the best exercise clothing, footwear and any other equipment you may need. There are also tips on setting goals and staying motivated while training.

You don't have to read the book from cover to cover in order to begin your training, although doing so will give

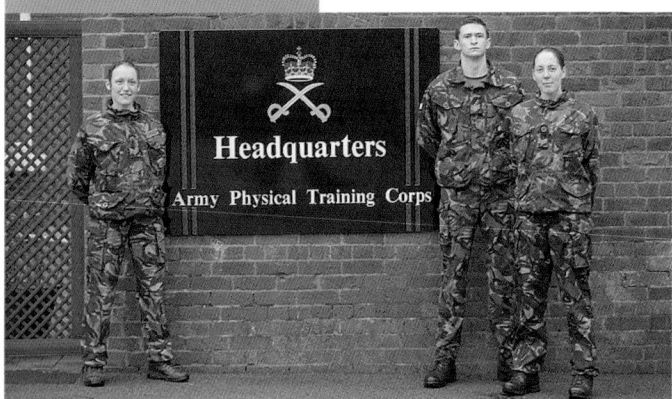

you the optimal preparation. If you already have a reasonable level of fitness, you can turn straight to the main programmes, which begin on page 124. However, do complete the questionnaire on page 112 to make sure it is safe for you to exercise and the fitness assessments on pages 113-117 so that you start at the right level. On page 121 you will find space to record and monitor the results of your assessments before, during and after you've completed the programmes. Turn to page 12 for a visual guide to the book. Good luck!

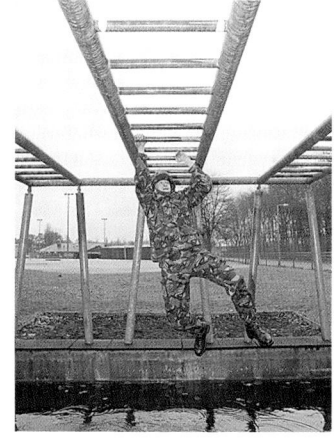
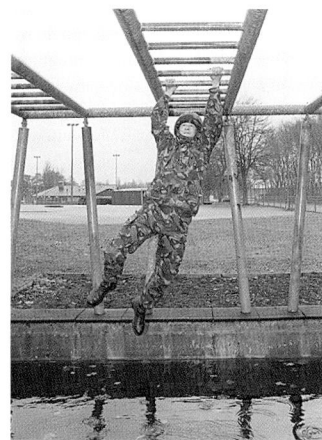

CAUTION

It is advisable to check with your doctor before beginning this or any strenuous exercise regime. Although every effort has been made to ensure the advice and exercise programmes in this book are safe and effective, the publishers and the Army do not accept any responsibility for injury or ill health that may arise from following them.

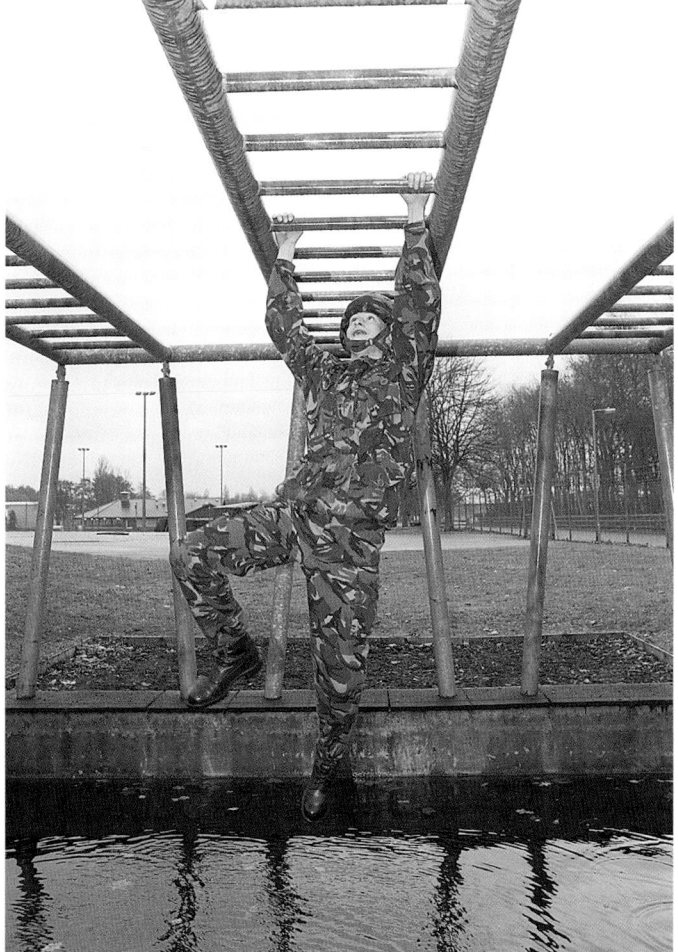

How to find what you need

PART 1

AEROBIC FITNESS (p.16)

STRENGTH (p.34)

PART 2

ASSESSING YOUR FITNESS LEVEL (p.112)

WHICH PROGRAMME IS RIGHT FOR YOU? (p.118)

PART 3

STAYING HEALTHY (p.150)

NUTRITION AND PERFORMANCE (p.156)

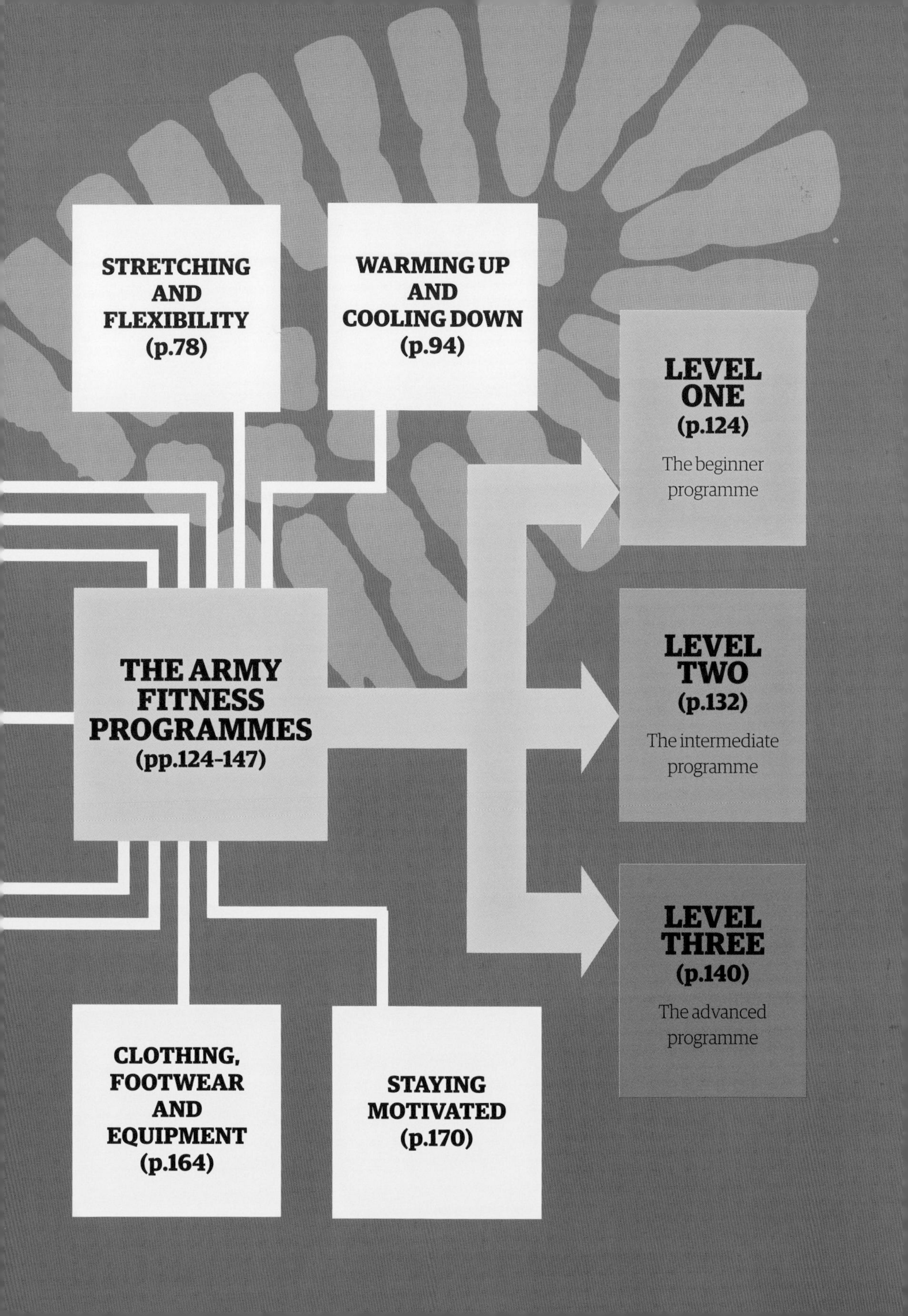

STRETCHING AND FLEXIBILITY (p.78)

WARMING UP AND COOLING DOWN (p.94)

LEVEL ONE (p.124)

The beginner programme

THE ARMY FITNESS PROGRAMMES (pp.124-147)

LEVEL TWO (p.132)

The intermediate programme

LEVEL THREE (p.140)

The advanced programme

CLOTHING, FOOTWEAR AND EQUIPMENT (p.164)

STAYING MOTIVATED (p.170)

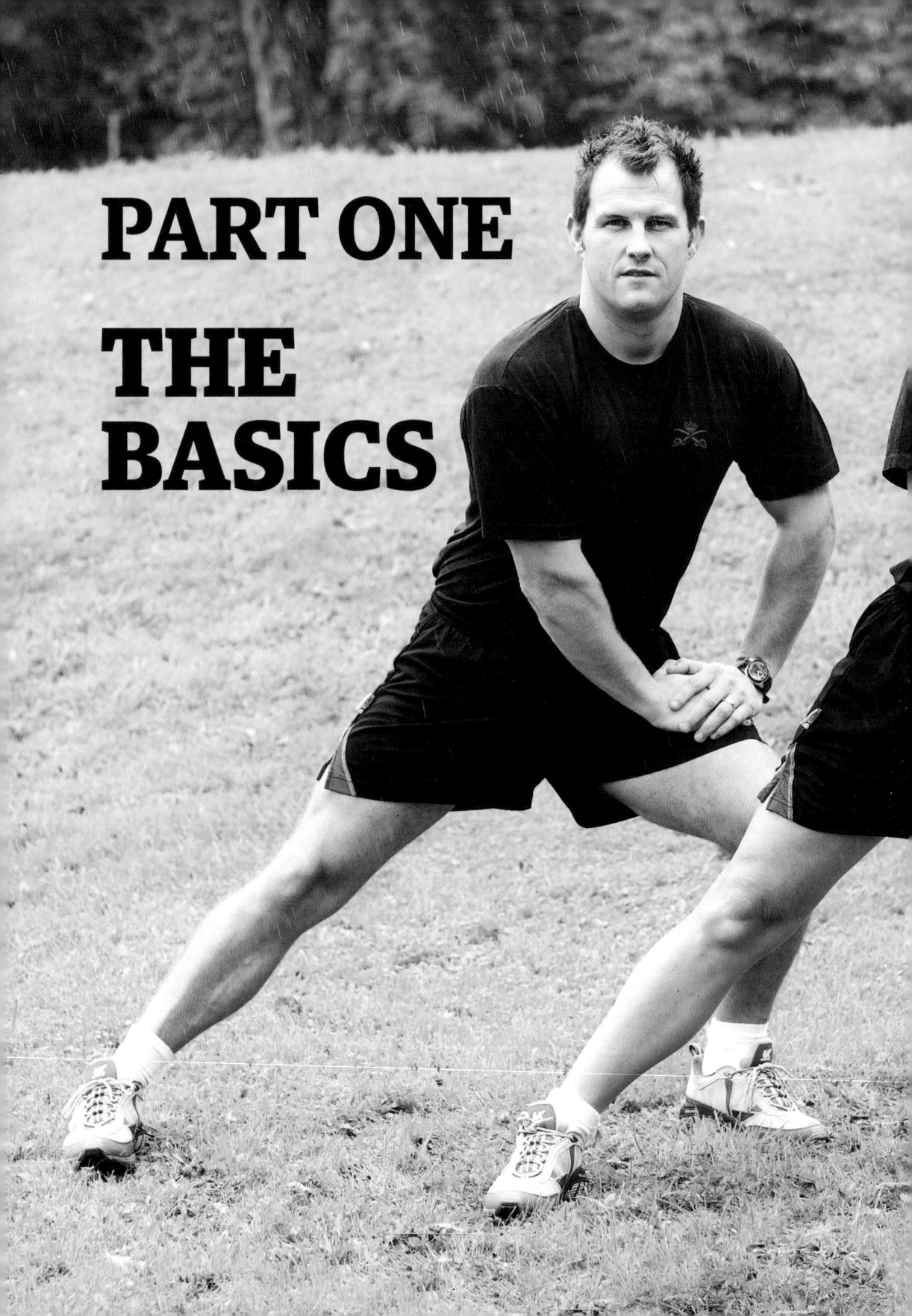

PART ONE

THE BASICS

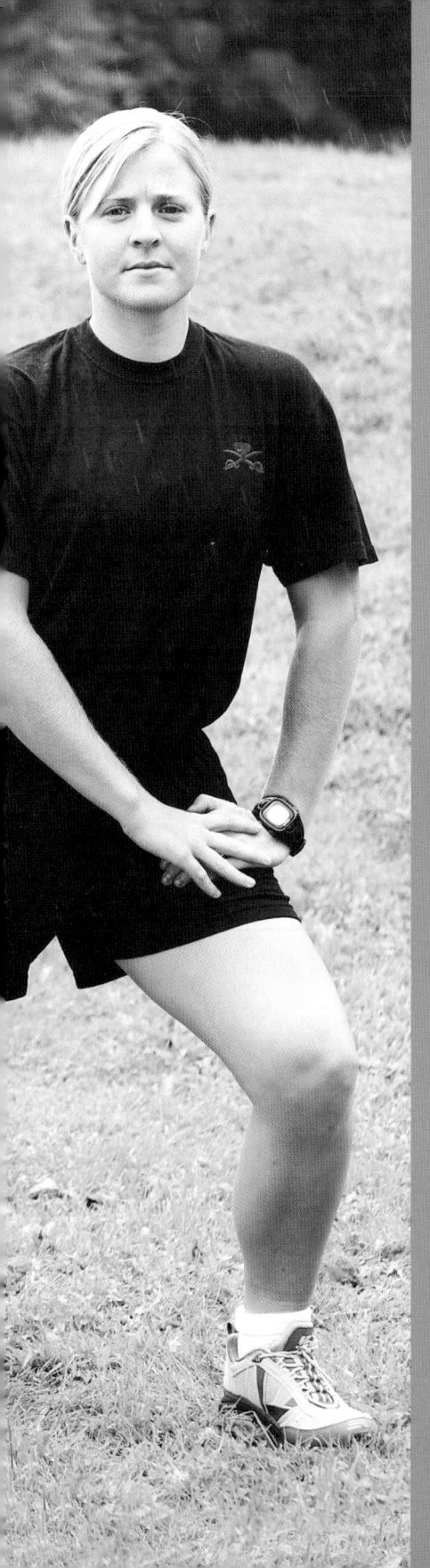

The Army has long recognised physical fitness as a fundamental requirement of every soldier. A good level of fitness ensures that soldiers can cope with the physical and psychological demands of the job, as well as reducing the time it takes for them to acclimatise to extreme conditions and recover from injury.

But why should you bother to get fit? Physical activity does a lot more than make you stronger, fitter and faster. It has an important role to play in improving many and varied aspects of health. Regular exercise can reduce the risk of cardiovascular disease, diabetes and hypertension - as well as having positive effects on everything from bone density to body fat levels and your psychological wellbeing. It can even help you live longer. This section looks at the three components of fitness - aerobic fitness, strength and flexibility - and how to improve and maintain them.

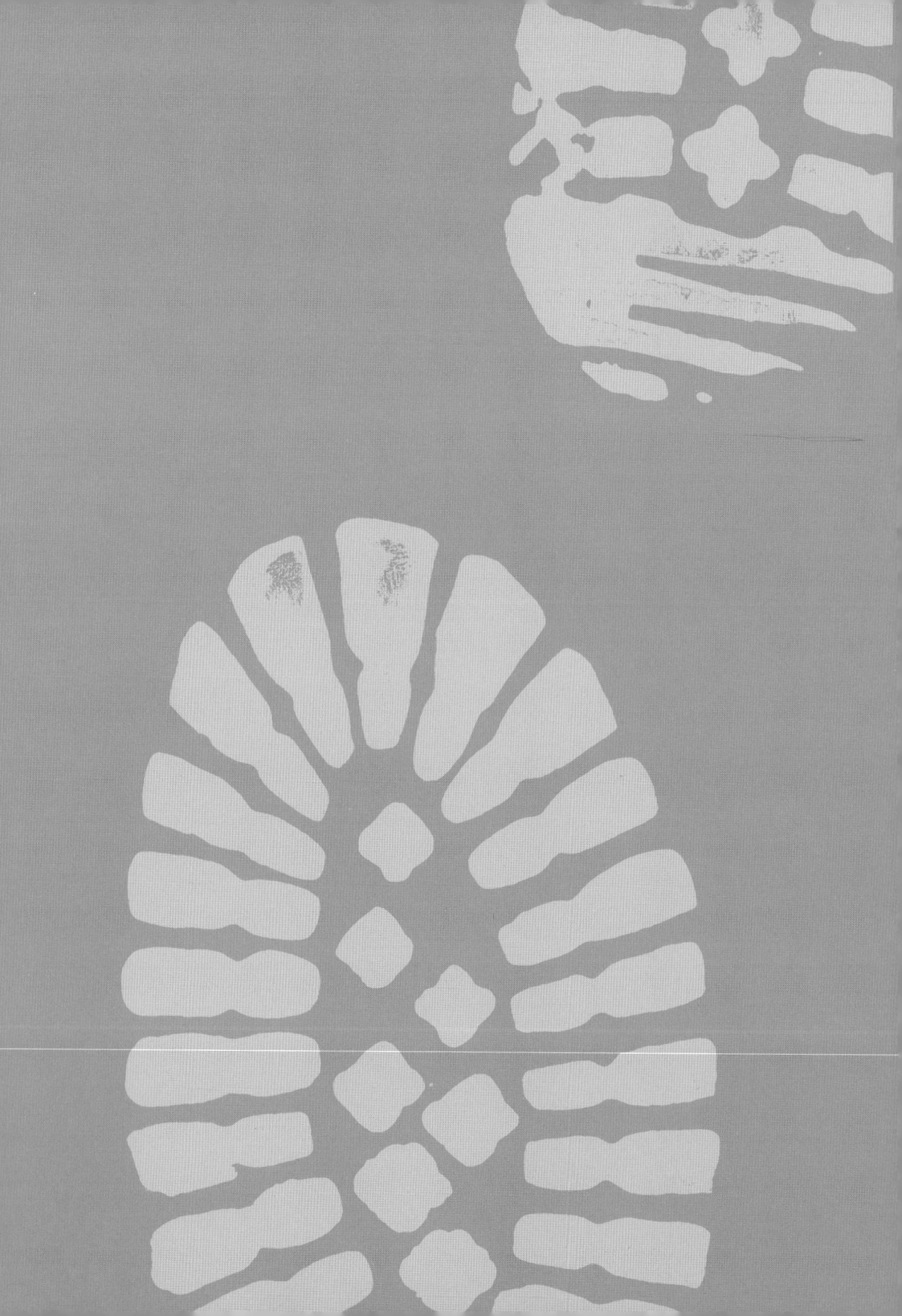

Aerobic fitness

What does being fit actually mean? The fitness of a footballer is very different from that of a gymnast, for example. The fitness of a martial artist cannot be compared to that of a marathon runner. Total fitness comprises a number of attributes, all of which have a different role to play in enhancing health, wellbeing and performance.

Aerobic or "cardiovascular" fitness (stamina) is concerned with the fitness of the circulatory and respiratory systems. Good aerobic fitness means that your heart, blood vessels and lungs can deliver sufficient oxygen and nutrients to your working muscles to enable you to keep going without fatigue for longer.

The official Army Fitness Programmes in Part Two (pp.124-147) are a great way of improving your aerobic fitness, but if you are new to aerobic exercise, try the four-week "start-up" programme at the end of this chapter first (pp.32-3), which will get you started safely. Once you have completed this, you should be ready to tackle the aerobic component of Level One of the Army Fitness Programmes (p.124).

Fit for anything

Aerobic exercise is the lynchpin of most physical activity programmes and, unsurprisingly, makes up a large part of the Army's physical training. Good aerobic fitness is integral to the performance of most physically demanding military tasks – whether it is marching all night, passing the Army's 2.4-km run test (p.116) or repeatedly moving boxes of heavy equipment. High levels of aerobic fitness are associated with improved military performance.

But the good news is that you do not need to conquer an Army obstacle course or run a marathon to reap the benefits. Brisk walking and cycling have been found to reduce the risk of heart disease and mortality.

Improving aerobic fitness

In general, cardiovascular or aerobic exercise involves using the body's large muscle groups, in a repetitive, rhythmic activity – such as walking or swimming – over a sustained period of time.

"Aerobic" means "with oxygen", and aerobic exercise must be performed at a level of intensity that enables your

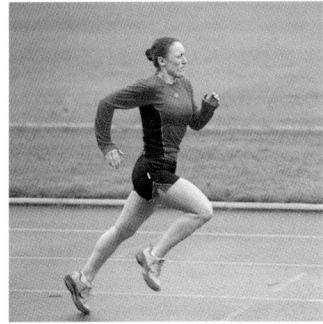

body to bring in enough oxygen to fuel demand. Many newcomers to exercise fall by the wayside because they immediately try to work at a high intensity which is difficult to sustain. If you try to exercise too vigorously, your body cannot take the required amount of oxygen in quickly enough and exercise soon becomes "anaerobic" (without oxygen). While this level of intensity has its benefits, you will only be able to sustain it for a very limited time, so it is not the best way to improve your aerobic fitness in the long term.

Activity can still take place over a broad spectrum of intensities, however, as shown in the table opposite. Walking is at the lower end of the scale, as it is an activity that you can continue for a prolonged period without too much effort. It is a 100% aerobic activity.

Further up the scale lie more challenging activities such as a tennis rally or a brisk run, which are harder to sustain for long periods. These are still mainly aerobic activities, with a small amount of anaerobic effort. And at the top end of the scale, you might have a 100-metre sprint, in which the effort is fully anaerobic.

Building a base

The secret to improving your aerobic fitness is to start by building a good base through working at a comfortable, sustainable level. When you have built a strong foundation, introduce more challenging activities that take you "outside your comfort zone".

A great way of increasing the intensity of your aerobic workouts is by interval training – mixing lower intensity aerobic exercise with bouts of harder effort. This allows you to introduce a challenge while still keeping the overall training load manageable. Mixing walking and running is a good way of trying interval training and is included in the start-up programme at the end of this chapter (pp.32–33).

HOW AEROBIC IS YOUR ACTIVITY?

This diagram shows the percentage contribution of aerobic and anaerobic energy supply for different activities.

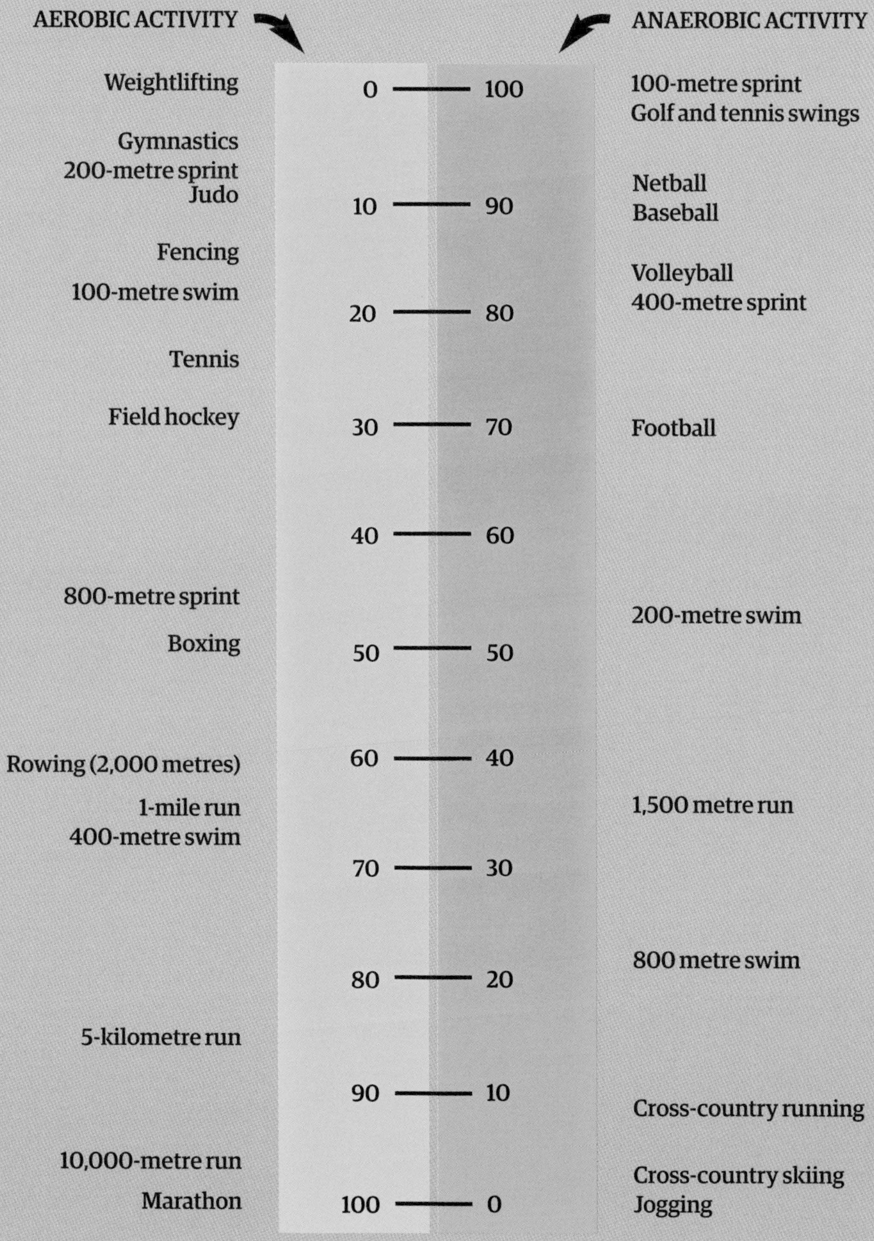

AEROBIC ACTIVITY			ANAEROBIC ACTIVITY
Weightlifting	0	100	100-metre sprint Golf and tennis swings
Gymnastics 200-metre sprint Judo	10	90	Netball Baseball
Fencing 100-metre swim	20	80	Volleyball 400-metre sprint
Tennis			
Field hockey	30	70	Football
	40	60	
800-metre sprint Boxing	50	50	200-metre swim
Rowing (2,000 metres)	60	40	
1-mile run 400-metre swim	70	30	1,500 metre run
	80	20	800 metre swim
5-kilometre run	90	10	Cross-country running
10,000-metre run Marathon	100	0	Cross-country skiing Jogging

The principles of training

There is more to training than simply getting out there and breaking a sweat. Effective training is underpinned by the following key principles.

Specificity means that the training you do has to be relevant to the goals you want to achieve. For example, a runner will not make great improvements in his 10-km time by playing golf. Specificity is especially important when it comes to gearing your fitness towards different sporting aims (such as running a race, or improving your tennis game) but it is less important when you are exercising to build all-round fitness.

Progressive overload means gradually increasing the level of difficulty of your physical activity programme. This is how you continue to get fitter. The Army uses a strategy known as "periodisation", which involves breaking the training period down into

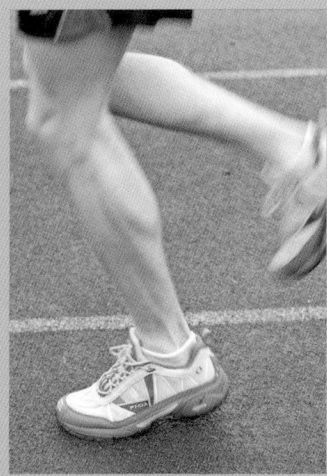

smaller chunks, each of which has a different focus, building on the one that came before. This ensures that progression is worked into the programme and that it occurs at a sensible rate.

The third principle is **adaptation**. It is only by placing the body under greater levels of stress than it is used to that it will undergo adaptation and grow stronger and more able to cope with greater physical demands. If you keep on doing the same workouts, time after time, without progression, you may soon hit a plateau in your fitness. However, if you increase your training

load too quickly or by too much, you will be at risk of over-training and may get injured.

If you follow the official Army Fitness Programmes in Part Two (pp.124-147) you will be able to progress at a safe and sensible rate by gradually increasing your training load and incorporating rest days to give you time to recover. It is while you are resting, not while you are training, that fitness adaptations take place. But do not overdo rest. The beneficial effects of training are reversible and will be lost if your rest periods are too long or your training load is too low.

You can manipulate your training load by altering the four elements that make up the **FITT** principle:

Frequency: how *often* you exercise.
Intensity: how *hard* you exercise.
Time: how *long* you exercise for.
Type: the *type* of exercise you do (for example, running, circuits).

Running

There are many ways of improving your aerobic fitness, but running is probably the simplest, most accessible option and is the most common form of endurance training in the Army. It is challenging but simple and you can do it anywhere, with very little equipment. Running also forms the basis of the Army Programmes (pp.124-147).

If you haven't run a step in years, then you should first turn to the four-week start-up programme at the end of this chapter (pp.32-33). This will take you from walking to running and help ease you into the main programmes.

If running isn't for you, there are plenty of other aerobic activities to try. Choose from walking, cycling, rowing or using the cardiovascular machines at the gym. See pages 28-31 for a guide to the most popular aerobic activities.

Why run?

There are many benefits to running, including:
- A reduced risk of heart disease.
- The loss of excess body fat through burning calories.

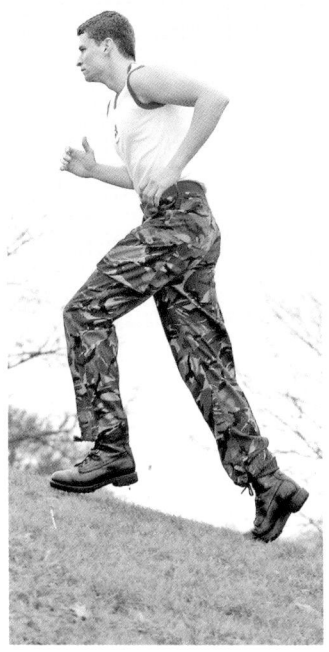

- An improvement in aerobic capacity.
- An increased resistance to fatigue.
- A strengthening of the ligaments and tendons in the lower body.
- A strengthening of the muscles of the lower body.

Everyone runs in a slightly different way, but there are a few general pointers worth knowing about, to make your running technique as smooth and efficient as possible. See page 22 for some tips on technique and body position.

DID YOU KNOW?

The most recent guidelines, produced jointly by the American College of Sports Medicine and the American Heart Association, recommend periods of moderately intense aerobic activity (such as walking) for 30 minutes or more, five days a week, or vigorously intense aerobic activity (such as running) for 20 minutes, three days a week (or a combination of the two types).

Light intensity "activities of daily living", such as walking around the home, shopping or casual walking of less than 10 minutes duration do not count towards the 30-minutes-a-day recommended amount. But more vigorous activities, such as heavy household chores, stair climbing and walking bouts of more than 10 minutes, can count towards the total.

How to run well

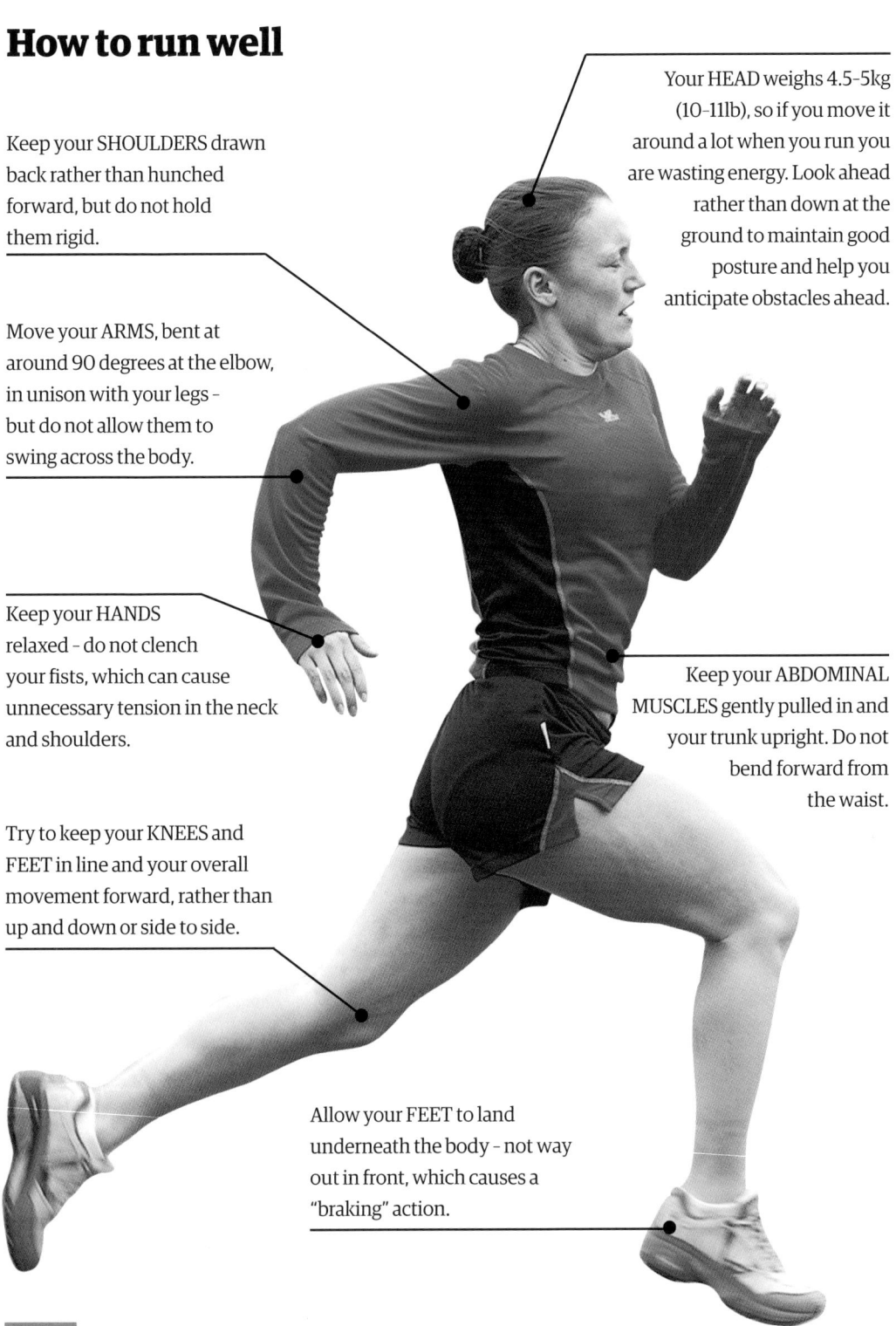

Keep your SHOULDERS drawn back rather than hunched forward, but do not hold them rigid.

Your HEAD weighs 4.5-5kg (10-11lb), so if you move it around a lot when you run you are wasting energy. Look ahead rather than down at the ground to maintain good posture and help you anticipate obstacles ahead.

Move your ARMS, bent at around 90 degrees at the elbow, in unison with your legs – but do not allow them to swing across the body.

Keep your HANDS relaxed – do not clench your fists, which can cause unnecessary tension in the neck and shoulders.

Keep your ABDOMINAL MUSCLES gently pulled in and your trunk upright. Do not bend forward from the waist.

Try to keep your KNEES and FEET in line and your overall movement forward, rather than up and down or side to side.

Allow your FEET to land underneath the body – not way out in front, which causes a "braking" action.

Running drills

A great way of improving your running technique is to introduce running drills into your training. Each drill hones in on one or two aspects of the running stride, allowing you to focus on that alone. Try the following drills over a distance of around 20 metres, repeating each one two or three times. You can incorporate them into your warm-up (pp.96-107) after you have raised your heart rate and loosened up.

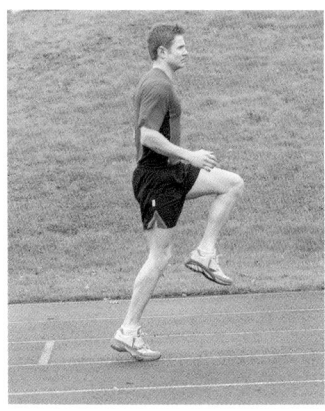

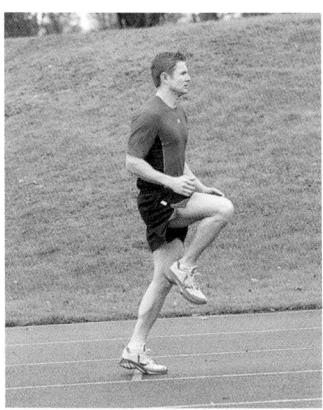

HIGH KNEES
From jogging, bring your knees up to hip height in front, without leaning back. This drill helps to get your foot landing below the knee rather than in front of it.

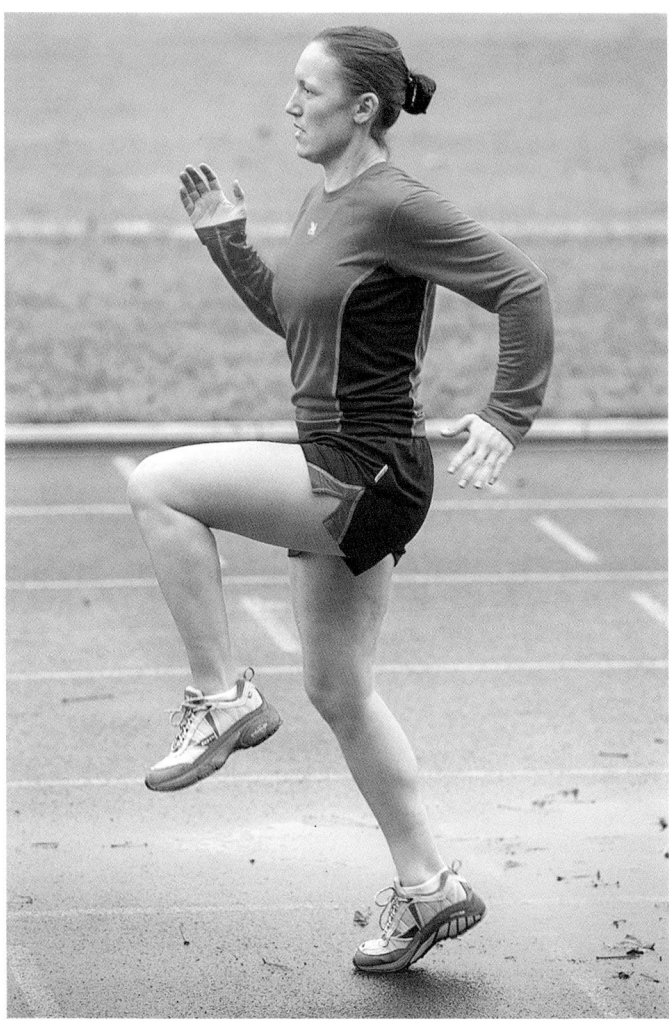

FAST FEET
Stand with feet together and then lift your feet quickly off the floor - as if you were running over hot coals. Travel forwards but focus on moving upwards. This drill will increase your stride rate.

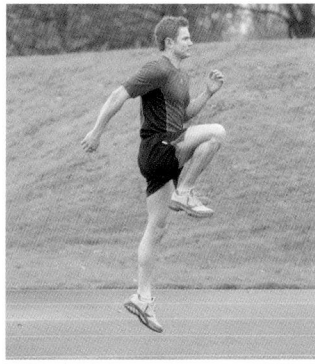

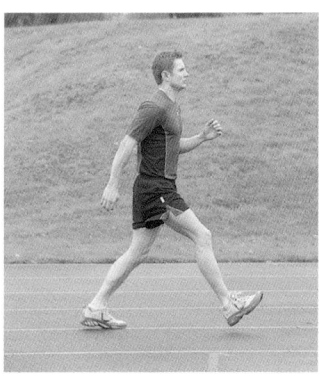

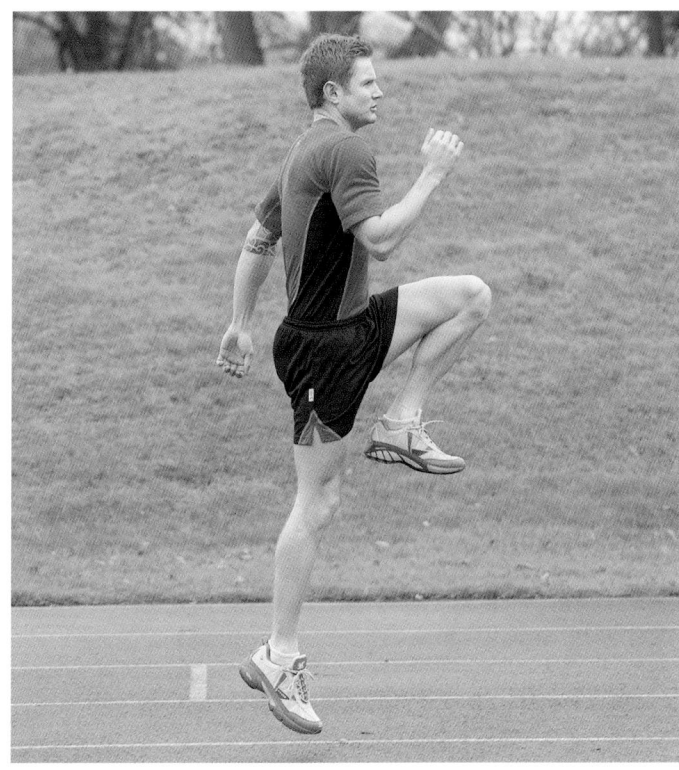

HIGH KNEE SKIPS

This is an exaggerated skipping motion. Skip forward on to one foot, lifting the knee high up in front, and using your arms in a running action. Aim for height as you skip from foot to foot. This drill improves power and glute strength (see p.41).

Stride rate

How fast you run is called your "stride rate", which is the combination of your stride length and stride frequency. The easiest way to work out your stride rate is to count the number of times your right foot lands during one minute of running. If you're in the region of 90 per minute (180 steps per minute in total), you're doing well. If your stride rate is considerably less than 90, concentrate on taking quicker, lighter steps, but remember to stay relaxed, and do not change your running action or the way your feet strike the ground.

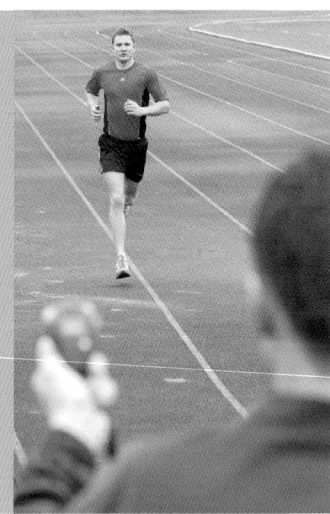

Run training

Jogging or running at a comfortable even pace – steady state running - will greatly improve your aerobic fitness and heart health and will also burn lots of calories. But think back to those principles of training outlined on page 20. Once steady jogging no longer poses a challenge, you know that it is time to increase the stakes by introducing some faster or tougher running. This doesn't mean that every run has to become an all-out sprint, it is just about interspersing a few more challenging sessions in among your steady-paced runs, in order to place new demands on your body and cause further fitness adaptations. Once you are comfortable running for 30 minutes or more, try introducing some of the following challenging sessions, which you will also find in the Army Fitness Programmes on pages 124-147.

Fartlek training

"Fartlek" is the Swedish word for speed play, and is a fun, unstructured way of progressing from steady running. This way of training entails running at different speeds, using landmarks such as trees or lampposts - or variations in the terrain - to increase or decrease pace. The duration and difficulty can be tailored to match ability. The Army also uses "Parlauf" or "pair running" in training, in which two runners take turns to set the pace. It keeps soldiers on their toes, as the runner at the back is the one who dictates the pace.

Interval training

Interval training means that your training includes faster bursts of effort interspersed with recovery jogging or rest. This means that you can work harder than normal, but only in limited bouts. Interval training is one of the most effective methods of elevating your fitness level. To ensure effectiveness, during the running interval you should be working hard enough to make talking difficult (see p.27).

The specific effects of interval training depend on:
■ The duration or distance of the work interval.
■ The pace of the effort.
■ The number of repetitions.
■ The duration of the jogging or rest interval.

DID YOU KNOW?

Running on softer surfaces, such as woodland trails, grass and sand – although more physically demanding – reduces the loading on one's joints and helps to prevent overuse injuries. It also improves strength and proprioception (awareness and stability) in the lower limbs. But take care when running on uneven surfaces and run in daylight, or in well-lit areas.

Hill running

When running up hills you are working against gravity, so you are improving leg strength as well as aerobic fitness. Hill reps (in which you repeatedly run up and then walk or jog down a particular hill) are a good way of introducing hill training to your regime. Aim for a short, quick stride with a good knee lift and maximum range of movement at the ankle. Running down hills is also good training, helping to strengthen the connective

Getting faster

The Army uses a number of techniques to improve running speed, including:

● **Sprint-assisted training drills**, such as downhill running and treadmill running, which help to increase stride frequency

● **Sprint-resisted training drills**, which include uphill running, running wearing weighted clothing or towing heavy objects, and running in sand or snow. These all increase strength, aerobic and muscular endurance.

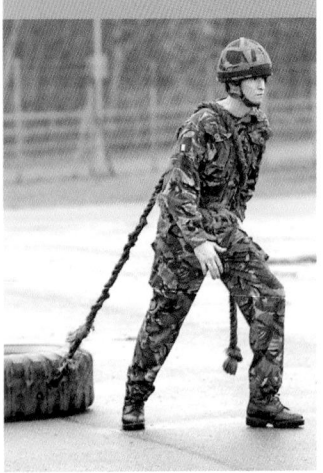

tissues and improve your stride rate and technique. But start on shallow slopes of not more than 10 degrees and only introduce downhill running gradually, to avoid muscle soreness. Hill training helps to:

■ Develop muscle elasticity.
■ Improve stride frequency.
■ Develop co-ordination, encouraging the proper use of arm action.
■ Improve muscular endurance.
■ Develop speed and strength.

Tempo running

Tempo running (or "threshold" running) is a continuous run performed at a brisk pace, just below the "lactate threshold" - the point

at which lactic acid builds up in the muscles faster than it can be cleared away. Working just below the threshold helps to push it up, so you can run faster without fatiguing. To start with, it is fine to break down tempo runs into stages.

How hard should it feel?

There are a few ways of measuring exercise intensity. One of the simplest is the "talk test":

■ When jogging or warming up you should be able to talk comfortably (known as "conversation pace").
■ On steady runs, you should be able to talk in short sentences.
■ On harder runs, your breathing should be heavy and it should be difficult to

say more than a few words at a time. Generally speaking, the shorter the bout of running, the harder the effort should be.

■ When performing maximal or near maximal efforts during interval or hill sessions you may be unable to get more than one word out at a time or only be able to say more than this with some difficulty.

WAYS TO RATE YOUR EXERCISE EFFORT

The "talk test" (left) is one simple way of measuring your level of effort when exercising. You can also use heart rate measured in beats per minute (BPM) as a guide to your level of physical exertion (see p.155), a Rate of Perceived Exertion (RPE) scale or a percentage effort scale.

The RPE and percentage effort scales refer to how hard you feel you are working and are given in the table below. The numbers relate to phrases used to rate how easy or difficult you find an activity. For example, 0 (nothing at all) would be how you feel when sitting in a chair; 10 (extremely hard) would be how you feel you are working during an exercise stress test or a very strenuous activity. In the programmes in Part Two (pp.124-147) a percentage effort rating is given, but if you prefer to use a different method, refer to this table to find an equivalent effort level using RPE or the talk test.

RPE scale	Effort (%)	How it feels	Talk test
0-1	0-10	Nothing at all	-
2	20	Just noticeable	-
3	30	Very light	-
4	40-50	Light	Could talk all day
5-6	50-60	Moderate	Converse comfortably
7	60-75	Moderately hard	Short sentences
8	75-80	Hard	Few words at a time
9	80-90	Very hard	One word at a time
10	90-100	Extremely hard	Difficulty talking

Other aerobic activities

While it is undoubtedly one of the best, running is not the only form of cardiovascular exercise. Walking, cycling, swimming and rowing are great complements, or alternatives, to running. They work your heart and lungs just as hard but without the repetitive impact of running and, because they use your muscles in a slightly different way, present new challenges. But remember, anything that gets your heart beating faster and makes you breathless counts as cardiovascular activity so this could include activities such as aerobics classes, circuit training and the gym stair climber. It is important to find an aerobic activity that you enjoy, so that you are likely to perform it regularly.

Cycling

The Army uses cycling and indoor cycling (spinning) to add variety to training and to help develop aerobic fitness to a high level. It is particularly effective for people who have not been active for some time, or soldiers who are injured, because the impact on the joints is lower. It is also a useful form of transport in the field and is often used in confined operational environments.

- Keep your upper body relaxed and regularly change hand position to avoid tension in your arms and shoulders.
- Keep your upper body and head still.
- Adjust your saddle height so that your hips stay level when you are pedalling.
- Maintain a constant pressure on the pedals all the way around the pedal stroke, rather than just pushing downwards.
- Keep your cadence (number of pedal strokes per minute) high rather than trying to push heavy gears slowly. This is more efficient.

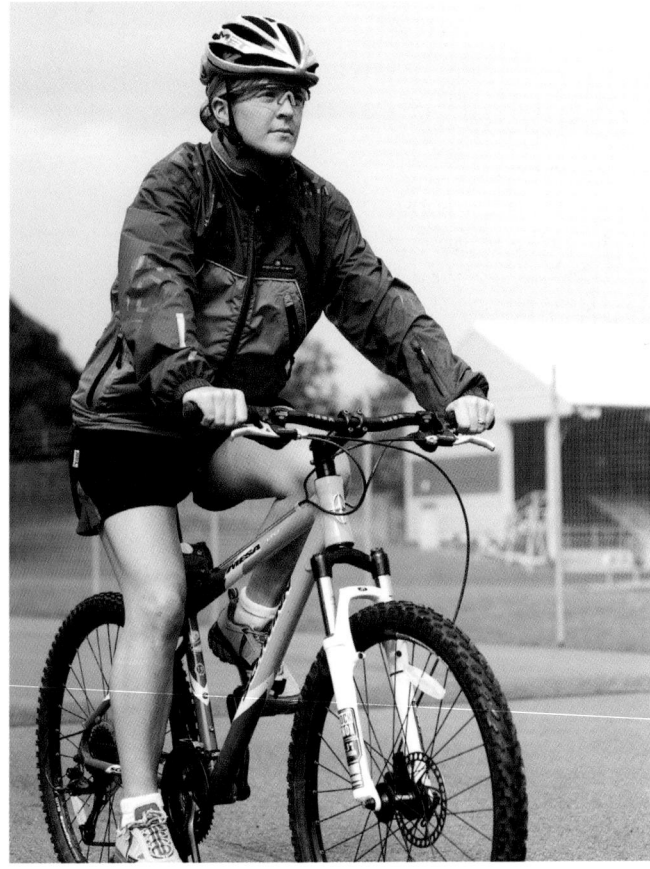

Swimming

Water-based exercise is widely used in the Army, from swimming and pool-based circuits or aerobics to hydrotherapy for rehabilitation. If you decide to make swimming your main form of aerobic activity, it is worth investing in a course of lessons to perfect your technique.

BREASTSTROKE

The main stroke used by the Army is breaststroke because it allows soldiers to see above the water line while they are swimming. It is also quieter than other strokes and easier to perform when wearing clothing. Breaststroke is a leg-dominant stroke, with around three-quarters of the effort coming from the lower body. When swimming breaststroke:

- Keep each stroke as long as possible. You will get faster by increasing the distance you travel with each stroke, not the number of strokes you make.
- Complete each stroke by bringing your feet together and do not pull with your arms until you have almost finished gliding.
- Keep your shoulders back and try to bring your

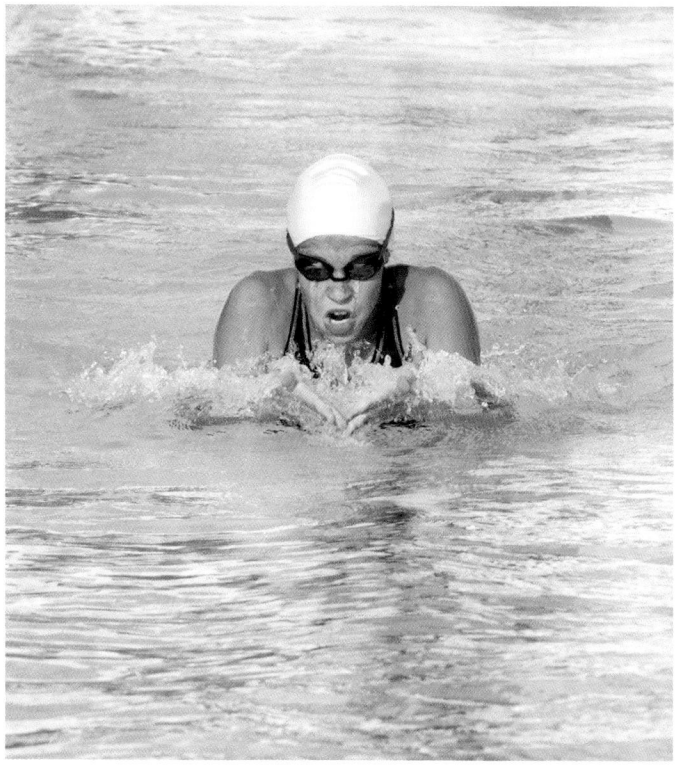

shoulder blades together at the end of the arm pull.
- Keep your abdominal muscles pulled in and do not overarch your back.
- Keep your hips high in the water, to avoid dragging your legs behind you.

FRONT CRAWL

Front crawl or "freestyle" is predominantly an upper body stroke - with the power coming from the back, shoulders and arms. It is a great stroke for fitness and distance swimming. When swimming front crawl:

- Do not swim flat in the water - roll your body from side to side.
- Make sure you finish off each stroke, bringing the hand out of the water after it brushes past your thigh and recovering the arm with a high elbow.
- Keep your head in line with your spine rather than craning your neck forward.
- Breathe out slowly when your head is in the water and, when you turn to breathe, only lift your head as far as you need to in order to clear the water.

Walking

Walking is a great form of moderate aerobic activity, suitable for almost anyone. It is also easy to fit into your day, as you probably already do at least some walking. It is merely a matter of looking for opportunities to increase the amount you currently do.

Many studies have clearly shown the health benefits of regular walking, leading to the recommendation that we each accrue 10,000 walking steps per day. Most of us fall short of that recommendation – 5,000 daily steps are more typical of today's sedentary population. But one failsafe way of increasing your steps is to start counting them. Research shows that wearing a pedometer – a simple device that you clip on to the waistband of your trousers and which records your step count over the course of the day – can increase your step count by 1,000 per day. Here are a few walking tips:

- Keep your head lifted, stomach pulled in and shoulders relaxed.
- Swing your arms naturally. Avoid carrying hand weights, since these put excessive stress on the elbows and shoulders.
- Do not overstride. Select a comfortable, natural step length.
- If you wish to move faster, take faster and shorter steps.

Rowing

As a highly demanding but low impact form of cardiovascular exercise, rowing is popular in the Army, with many soldiers competing in indoor competitions using rowing machines.

Rowing works most of the body's major muscle groups including the legs and bottom, back and shoulders. It is also one of the few aerobic activities where the

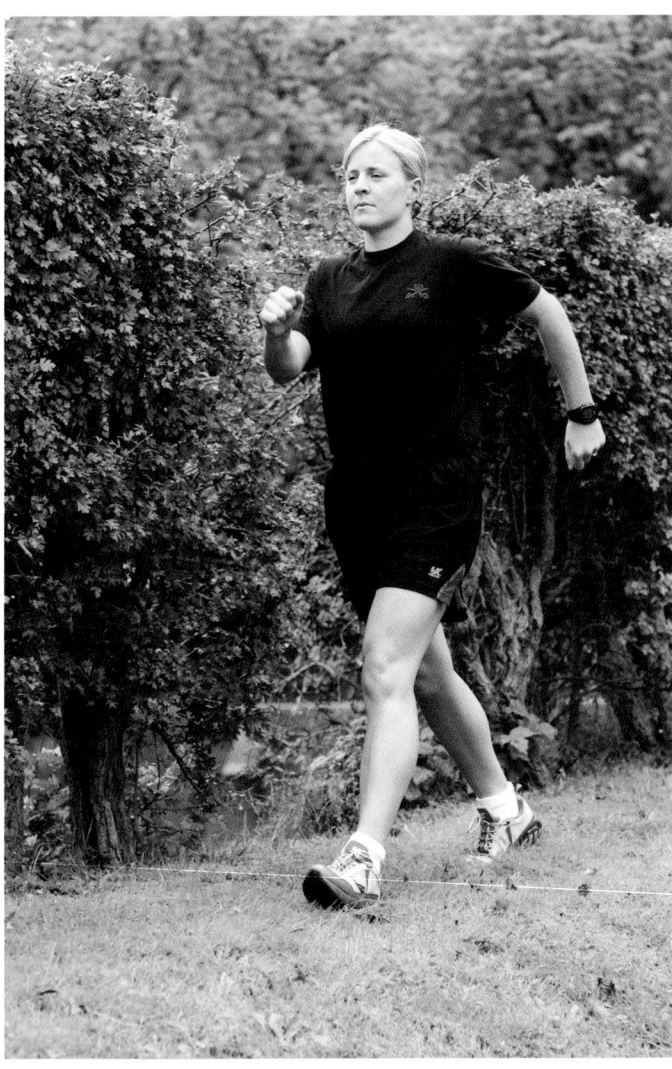

effort comes from pulling backwards rather than pushing forwards, which is beneficial to posture. Here are a few tips for rowing:

■ Keep your back straight throughout the stroke.

■ Initiate the pull with your legs, before pulling with your arms.

■ Do not "lock out" your knees and elbows when they are extended.

■ Engage the shoulder blades as you take your arms behind you.

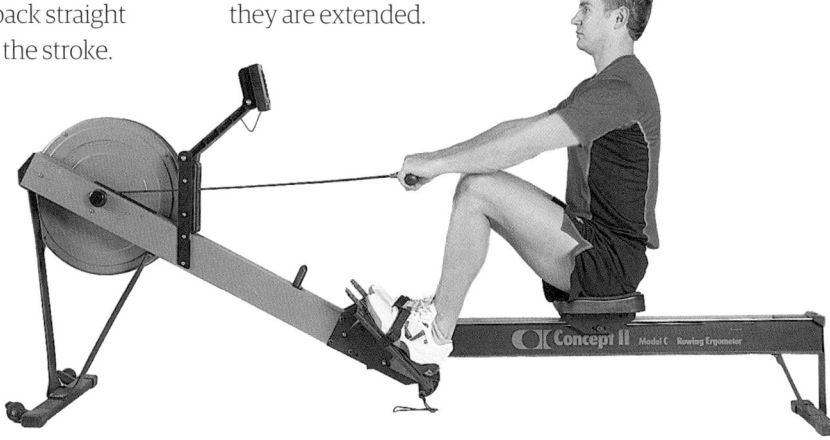

Aerobic activity for weight loss

There is little doubt that aerobic activity is integral to maintaining a healthy weight. However, the amount needed for successful weight loss appears to be higher than that needed to derive other health benefits. The good news, however, is that while vigorous exercise generally bestows greater health benefits than moderate intensity exercise, this is not the case with weight loss, where both levels have an equal effect, providing the overall amount of energy expenditure is the same. In other words you get the same weight-loss benefits from working at a low intensity for a long time as you do from working at a high intensity for a short time. The other important message as far as aerobic activity and weight loss are concerned is that it seems that a combination of leisure-time physical activity and designated exercise (workouts) is the best way of maximising calorie expenditure.

Research by the US National Weight Control Registry found that successful weight loss maintenance entailed burning 400 calories per day through exercise while a study in the *Journal of the American Medical Association* found that in a group of overweight women who embarked on a diet and exercise programme, 40 minutes every day produced and maintained substantial weight loss. Smaller amounts of activity did not succeed in keeping the weight off.

Four-week aerobic fitness start-up programme

This programme introduces you to running, so that you will be ready to tackle the aerobic component of the official Army Fitness Programmes in Part Two (pp.124-147). Aim to complete all four sessions each week, on non-consecutive days where possible. These "rest days" give your body a chance to recover and adapt, so do not be tempted to sneak in extra sessions. If you are already fairly aerobically fit you can skip this programme and go straight to Part Two. If you have been sedentary for a while you may need to repeat a week or two of this programme before progressing to the next week. Start each session with a warm-up and finish with a cool-down (pp.96-109).

DID YOU KNOW?

Aerobically fit individuals have a 25-50% lower overall risk of developing cardiovascular disease and a 42% lower risk of type 2 diabetes than those who are not aerobically fit.

Effort levels

- During the run segments, you should be working at approximately 50-60% effort (see p.27 for a reminder of how hard these different effort levels should feel).
- During the walk recoveries, aim for 30% effort.
- Brisk walking should be at approximately 40-50% effort.

Session

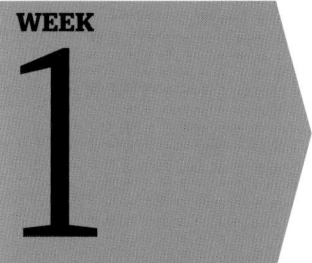

WEEK 1

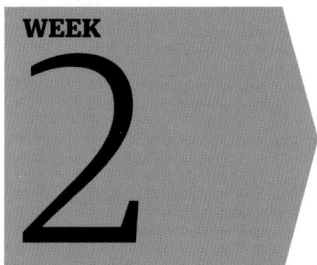

WEEK 2

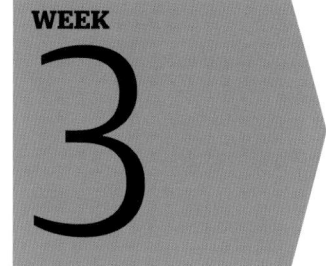

WEEK 3

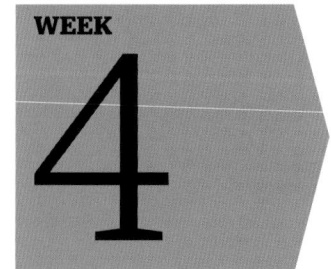

WEEK 4

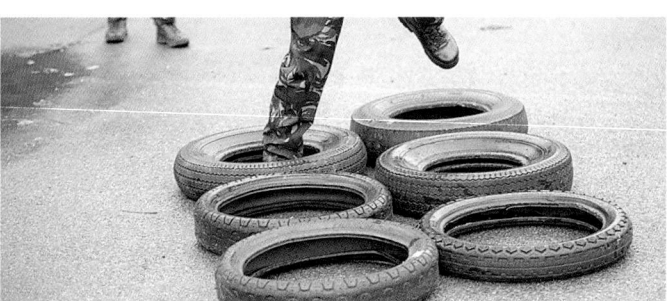

DAY 1		DAY 2		DAY 3		DAY 4
● Run 1 min ● Walk 3 mins Repeat x 4	REST DAY	● Run 1 min ● Walk 3 mins Repeat x 5	REST DAY	● Run 1 min ● Walk 3 mins Repeat x 4	REST DAY	● 20-min brisk walk
● Run 2 mins ● Walk 3 mins Repeat x 4	REST DAY	● Run 2 mins ● Walk 3 mins Repeat x 5	REST DAY	● Run 2 mins ● Walk 3 mins Repeat x 4	REST DAY	● 25-min brisk walk
● Run 3 mins ● Walk 2 mins Repeat x 4	REST DAY	● Run 3 mins ● Walk 2 mins Repeat x 5	REST DAY	● Run 3 mins ● Walk 2 mins Repeat x 4	REST DAY	● 30-min brisk walk
● Run 4 mins ● Walk 2 mins Repeat x 5	REST DAY	● Run 5 mins ● Walk 2 mins Repeat x 4	REST DAY	● Run 4 mins ● Walk 2 mins Repeat x 5	REST DAY	● Walk 10 mins ● Jog 10 mins ● Walk 10 mins

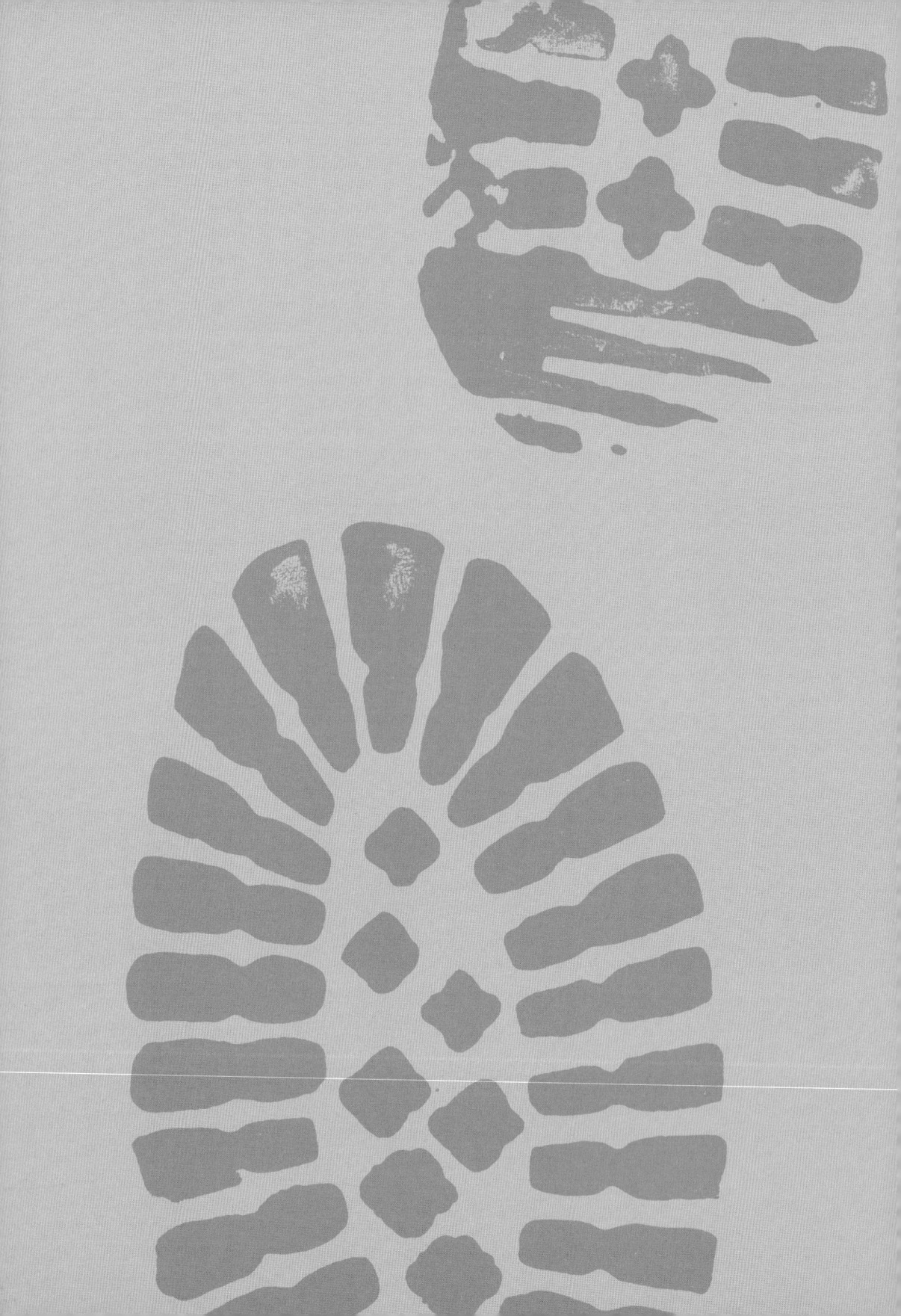

Strength

Getting stronger can have a positive effect on many aspects of your life and health, even if you do not spend your days lifting and carrying heavy equipment, like many soldiers do.

Daily activities – from gardening and moving furniture, to climbing the stairs – become easier and less tiring when your muscles are strong and more resistant to fatigue. Improved strength will also enhance your appearance, because muscles get firmer when they are strengthened, giving you a more defined, toned body shape. Strength or "resistance" training also offers major health benefits. Research published in the *Journal of the American Heart Association* indicates that such training can favourably affect many risk factors for heart disease, including cholesterol levels, blood pressure, glucose metabolism and body composition (the ratio of muscle to fat), as well as boosting bone density.

If you are fairly new to strength training, the four-week "start-up" programme at the end of this chapter (pp.76-77) will get you going. Once you have completed this, you should be ready to tackle the strength component of the Level One Programme (p.124).

How strength training works

Strength is all about exerting a force. When muscles exert a force, they pull on bones, to enable movement to occur or a position to be maintained. To make muscles stronger, therefore, you should progressively "overload" them with a weight or other form of resistance. Provided the right level and type of overload is placed upon the muscles, and this is done often enough, they will adapt to the challenge by getting stronger.

While some strength training exercises target one major muscle group (isolation exercises), others call upon multiple muscle groups simultaneously. These are called "compound" exercises and are generally held to be more "functional" than isolation exercises, as in everyday activities, we tend to use our muscles in groups rather than in isolation.

The Army favours compound moves in their exercise programmes, but you can supplement these with exercises that hone in on specific areas of the body.

Reps, sets and the rest

The specific way you train muscles determines the type of strength they develop. An ability to contract repeatedly prior to fatigue is referred to as **muscular endurance** while an ability to contract a muscle group forcefully just one or a few times is referred to as **muscular strength**. **Power** is the ability to exert force at speed.

There are three factors you can manipulate to influence training outcomes. Firstly, the **number of times** you do an exercise (known as repetitions, or "reps"). Secondly, the **number of sets** you do (a set is a pre-determined number of repetitions performed

PTI Tip

Make sure you balance "pushing" exercises with "pulling" ones, to avoid muscular imbalance.

consecutively) and, finally, the **amount of rest** you take in between sets.

In the Army, the staple is three sets, but you might use anything between 1-5 sets, depending on the specific aim and purpose of the session. If you are new to strength training, initially a single set will produce results - but you will progress more quickly if you do three or more sets.

If you are a beginner, as a starting point aim to perform 10 repetitions per set. That means lifting a weight, or performing the exercise, 10 times - using a resistance level that makes the last couple of repetitions difficult. If the last couple of reps feel easy, use a heavier weight or a harder exercise. Follow these tips to make the most of your strength training:

■ **Focus on muscular endurance** by increasing your repetitions but use less weight or go for an easier exercise option.

■ **Focus on strength and size** by using fewer reps but an increased level of weight or a more challenging exercise.

■ **Focus on power** (a product of strength and speed) by performing the exercises more explosively, or at a faster pace, but without reducing the level of resistance significantly. (Use fewer reps than you would for muscular endurance.)

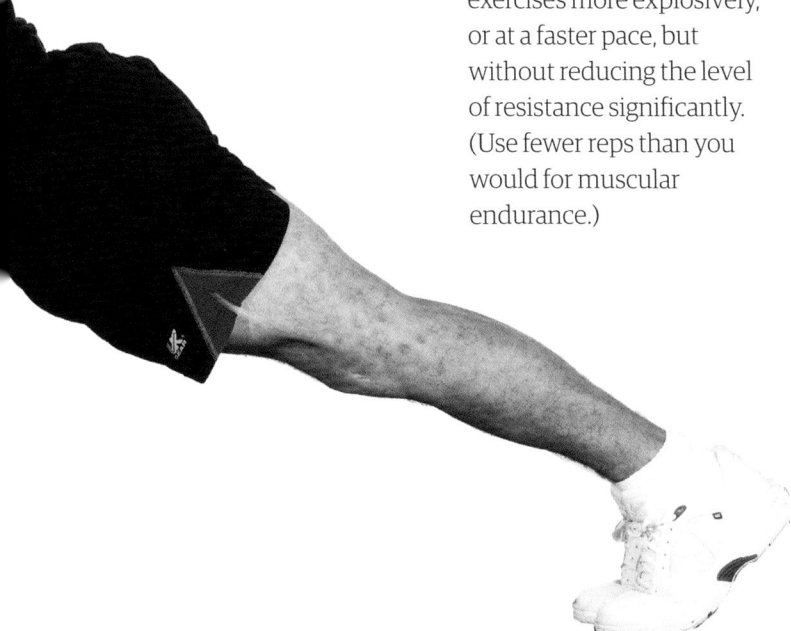

■ Initially, **rest for one to two minutes** between each set to allow the muscles to recover before they have to work again. If you want to focus on endurance, rest for a shorter period. If you want to focus on strength, rest for a longer period.

■ **To see results**, two to three sessions per week is ideal.

What muscles should we train?

Many of us have a tendency to train only the muscles we can see in the mirror. But for a balanced, well-proportioned body which functions efficiently, we must train the whole body and target muscle groups in a number of different ways. For example, to fully work the trunk region, you need to have a wider repertoire of exercises than sit-ups. That is not to say sit-ups don't have a place in your programme – in fact, the two-minute sit-up test (p.115) is one of the principle Army muscular endurance tests. But the more trunk muscles you work, and the more angles you work them from, the better the results will be.

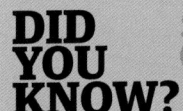

DID YOU KNOW?
Research shows that muscles in the upper body respond to strength training more quickly than those in the lower body. So you can see results in the top half more quickly.

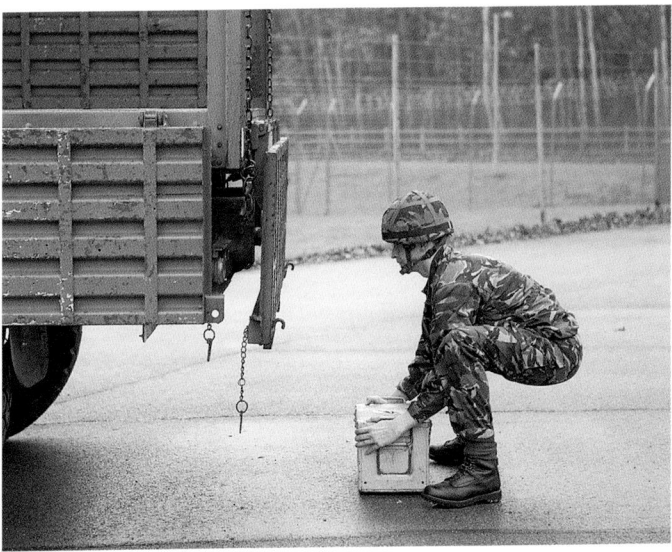

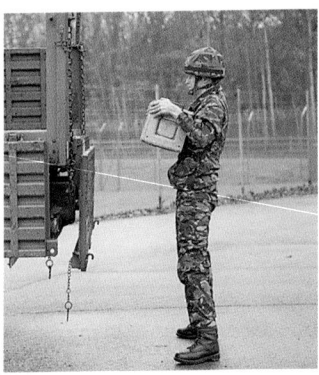

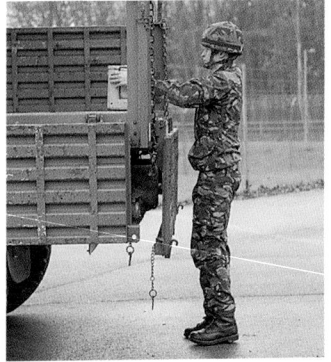

A strong, well-balanced mid-section is not just aesthetically pleasing. This area (incorporating the abs and back) is instrumental in practically all sports and physical performance. It is also crucial in maintaining good posture and preventing injury even when you are not involved in sports.

A fit and strong upper body is not only vital for lifting and carrying heavy weights such as ammunition boxes, it also contributes to better sports performance.

The muscle groups of the lower body are among the largest of all. They include the gluteals, quadriceps and calves (pp.39–41). These muscles are the foundation for most physical activities, from running and marching to pivoting and kicking.

The BICEPS run along the front of the upper arm, and bend the elbow.

The RECTUS ABDOMINIS or "six pack" muscle runs along the front of the stomach, from the sternum to the pubic bone. It flexes the trunk forwards and assists with lateral flexion (to the side).

The HIP FLEXORS sit on the front of the hip and bend (flex) the hip.

The DELTOID muscle group cups the shoulder area, allowing pushing, pulling and lifting motions, each of which focuses on a different part of the muscle group.

The PECTORALS or "pecs" span the chest area and facilitate "pushing" motions with the arms, as in a press-up.

The QUADRICEPS or "quads", covering the front of the thigh, mainly serve to extend the knee joint (such as in running or jumping).

PTI Tip

When working with weights, it is a good idea to perform a few "warm-up" reps without the weights first, or with light weights, to prepare yourself.

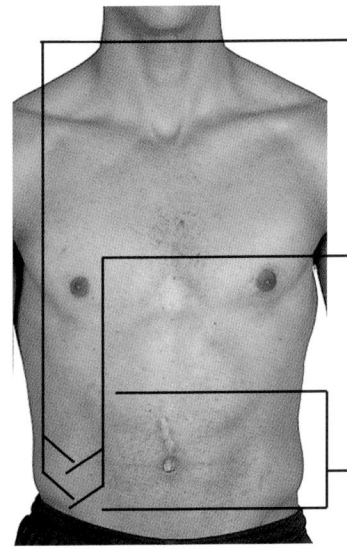

The EXTERNAL OBLIQUES sit along the side of each side of the waist. They flex the trunk to the same side, and rotate it to the opposite side. (For example, the external obliques on the right flex the trunk to the right and rotate the trunk to the left). They also assist with forward flexion.

The INTERNAL OBLIQUES sit below the external obliques, and their fibres run in the opposite direction. They flex and rotate the trunk to their own side. (For example, the internal obliques on the right flex and, in conjunction with the external obliques on the left, rotate the trunk to the right.)

The TRANSVERSUS ABDOMINIS muscle is a deep-set "corset" of muscle that wraps around the trunk from the belly button to the spine. Its main action is to compress and flatten the abdomen.

The ERECTOR SPINAE muscles are situated along the entire length of the spine, and serve to extend it. They also assist in lateral flexion of the spine.

The MULTIFIDUS muscles lie beneath the erector spinae, along each side of the spinal column, and are important spinal stabilisers. They also help to extend the spine and to rotate it to the opposite side from their position.

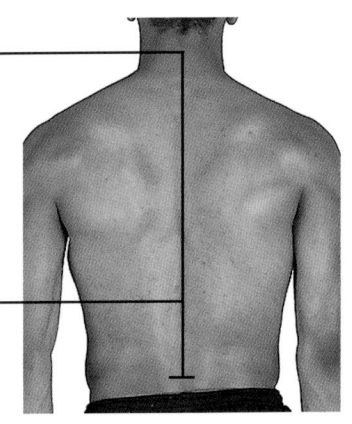

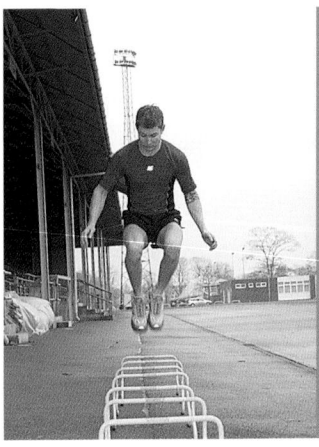

Power up

Power is the ability to exert force at speed. For example, lifting your body weight off the ground in an explosive jump. Training to improve your power involves adding an element of explosiveness to exercises (for example, a squat jump, in which your feet leave the ground between reps). However, it is not advisable to use this type of exercise until you have built a good grounding with more general strength training, as the risk of injury is greater.

The RHOMBOID and TRAPEZIUS muscles are situated in the middle of the upper and middle back and draw the arms and shoulder blades backwards, as in rowing.

The large LATISSIMUS DORSI span the entire back from the shoulders to the base of the spine in a "fan" shape.

The TRICEPS along the back of the upper arm straighten the arm at the elbow.

The QUADRATUS LUMBORUM muscle sits towards the back of each side of the waist and is an important muscle in stabilising the pelvis and spine. It also flexes the trunk to the same side and "hitches" the hip by elevating the pelvis.

The HAMSTRINGS, along the back of the thighs, work to bend the knee and help extend the hip.

The GLUTEALS or "glutes" are the powerful muscles of the bottom and hips, which work to extend the hip, rotate it or "abduct" it, as in when the leg is lifted out to the side.

The CALVES in the lower legs work to raise the body on to the toes (plantar flexion) and are heavily called upon during activities such as running, jumping, hopping and stretching to reach high places.

DID YOU KNOW?
Improving your leg strength reduces the time each foot spends on the ground during running by 0.02 seconds. That could take a full minute off your 1.5-mile time.

The Army exercises

Convinced that strength training is worth the effort? Well the good news is you don't need to spend hours in the gym honing your muscles to get results. The following 15 exercises are all used by the Army in physical training and are the moves that feature in the 12-week Army Fitness Programmes (pp.124-147).

For each one, easier and tougher options are indicated where possible, to suit your level of ability. If you want to work harder on specific body areas, as well as add interest, you can supplement these exercises with the additional exercises that target those areas on pages 64 to 75.

Upper body exercises

1 PRESS-UP

Soldiers do a lot of press-ups – they are a key element of military physical training. To do them correctly, begin with arms approximately shoulder-width apart, fingers facing forward, back straight and body in a straight line. Look slightly ahead, not at the floor. (This is to simulate the fact that you would need to keep looking ahead while moving forward in a combat situation.)

Lower your body towards the floor, elbows pointing back not splaying out to the side. Stop when your chest and hips are an inch off the floor, and then straighten the arms to return to the start position. That counts as one rep.

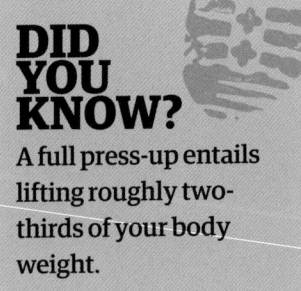

DID YOU KNOW?

A full press-up entails lifting roughly two-thirds of your body weight.

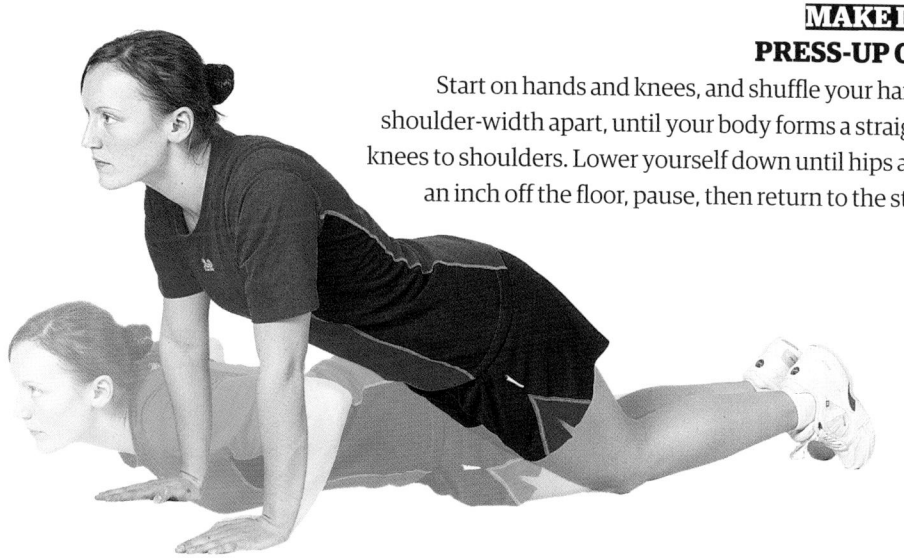

MAKE IT EASIER
PRESS-UP ON KNEES

Start on hands and knees, and shuffle your hands forward, shoulder-width apart, until your body forms a straight line from knees to shoulders. Lower yourself down until hips and chest are an inch off the floor, pause, then return to the start position.

MAKE IT EASIER
INCLINE PRESS-UP

Adopt the full press-up position, as outlined above, but this time place your hands on a raised surface (the higher the surface, the easier the exercise) rather than the floor. Lower your chest and hips towards the support, keeping your body in a straight line.

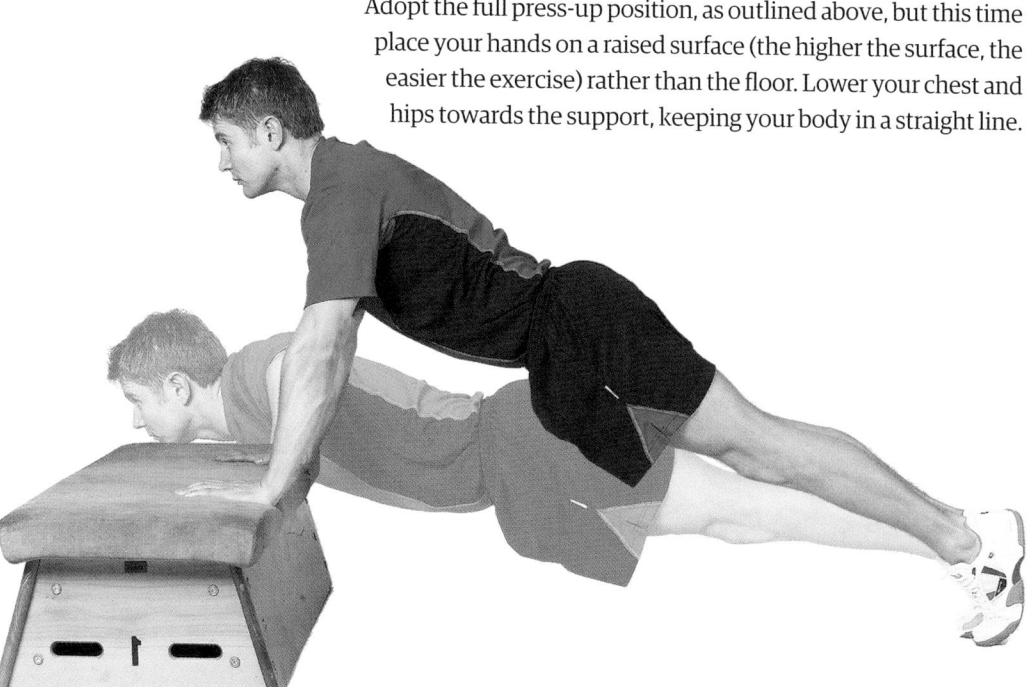

PTI Tip

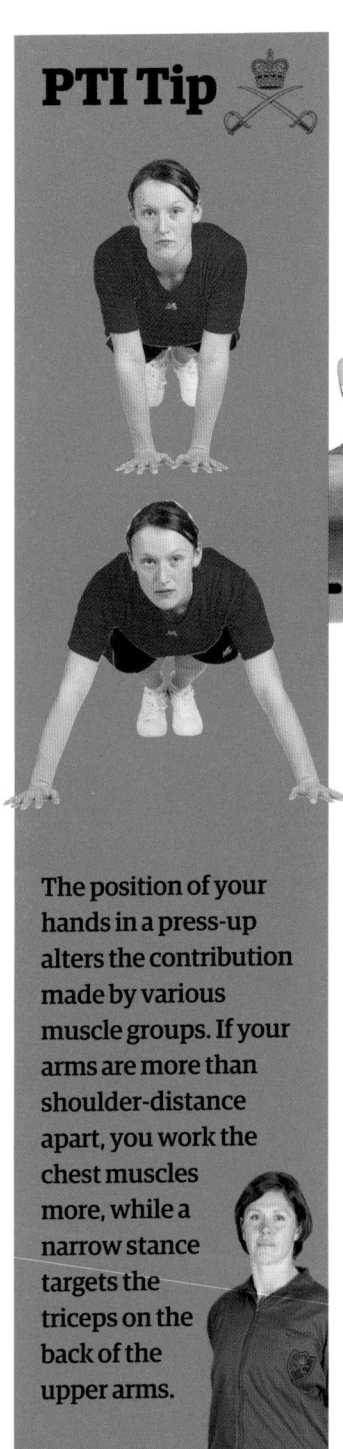

The position of your hands in a press-up alters the contribution made by various muscle groups. If your arms are more than shoulder-distance apart, you work the chest muscles more, while a narrow stance targets the triceps on the back of the upper arms.

MAKE IT HARDER
DECLINE PRESS-UP

OK with the Army issue press-up? Now try it with your feet placed on a raised surface, such as a chair, rather than on the floor – so that your shoulders and head are lower than your hips. Perform full press-ups as normal.

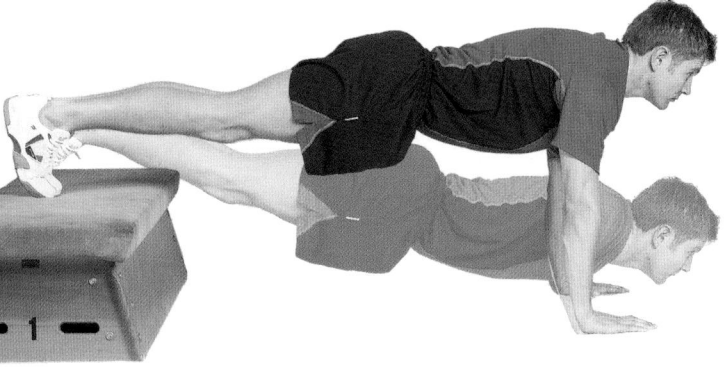

MAKE IT HARDER
CLAP PRESS-UP

Another way of making press-ups harder is to take your hands away and clap between each repetition.

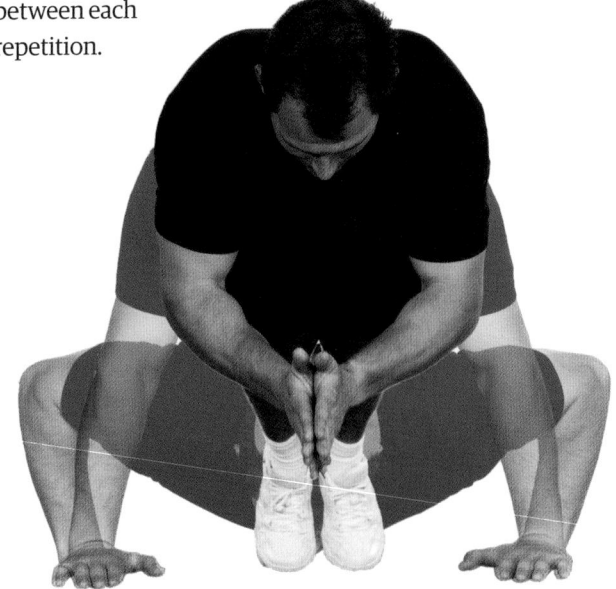

② PULL-UP

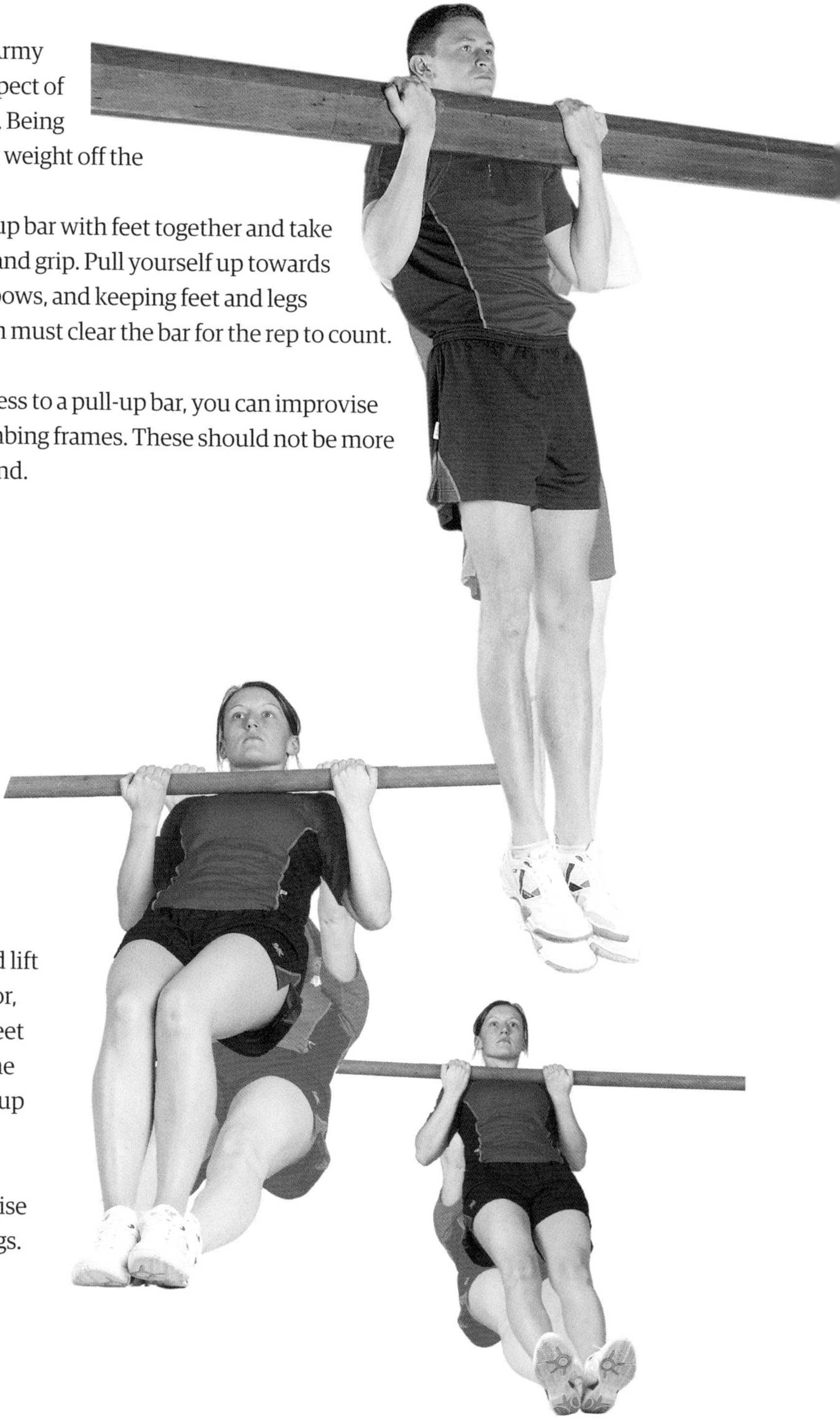

Pull-ups (or "heaves"' in Army speak) are another key aspect of military physical training. Being able to lift your own body weight off the ground is a crucial skill.

Stand beneath a pull-up bar with feet together and take hold of it with an underhand grip. Pull yourself up towards the bar, bending at the elbows, and keeping feet and legs locked together. Your chin must clear the bar for the rep to count. Slowly lower and repeat.

If you do not have access to a pull-up bar, you can improvise with tree branches or climbing frames. These should not be more than five feet off the ground.

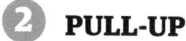

MAKE IT EASIER
PULL-UP WITH BROOMSTICK AND TWO CHAIRS

Place a broomstick over two sturdy chairs that are placed close together.

Take hold of the broomstick with an underhand grip, arms shoulder-width apart, and lift your body clear of the floor, keeping knees bent and feet on the floor. Then bend the elbows to bring the chest up towards the broomstick.

Pause then lower and repeat. To make the exercise harder, straighten your legs.

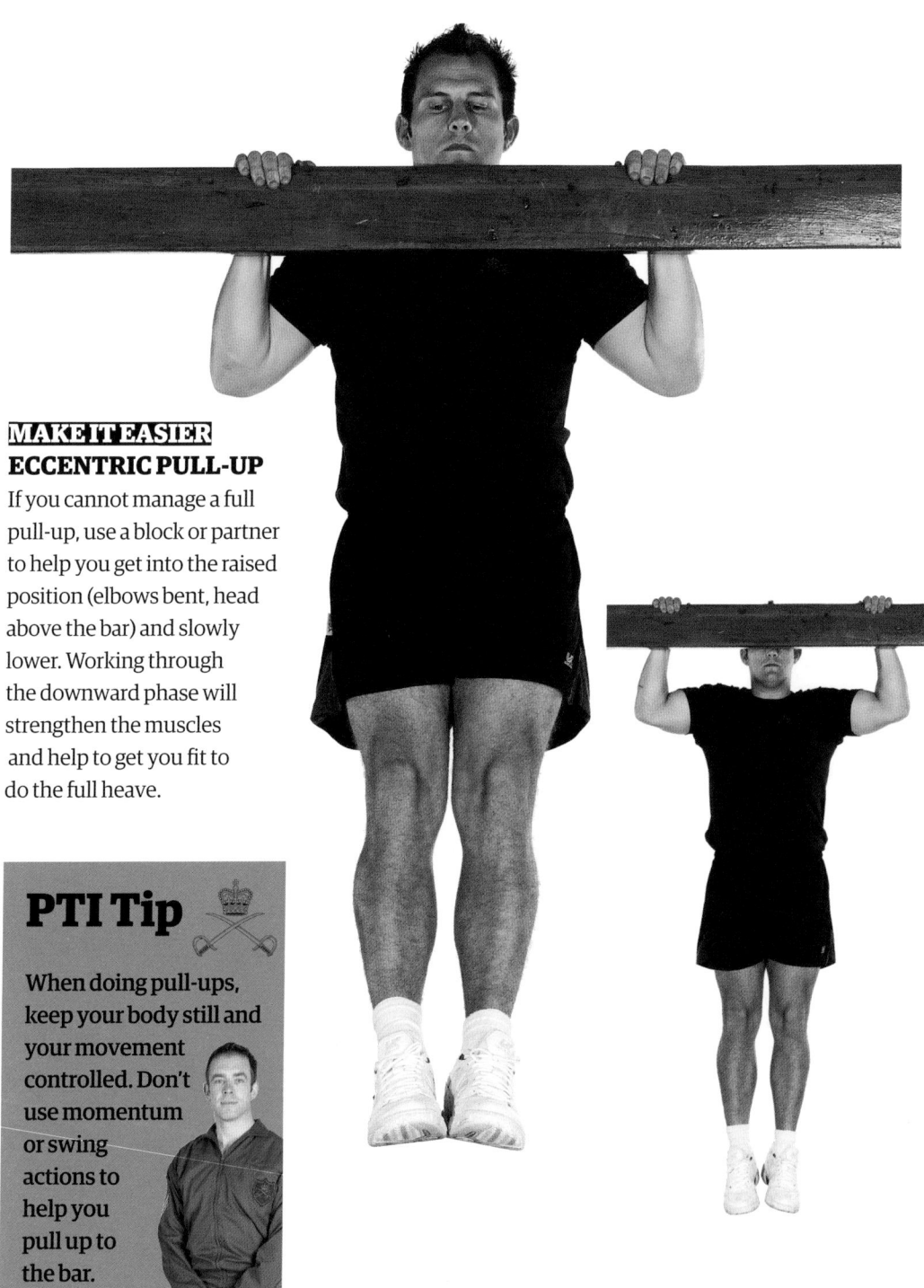

MAKE IT EASIER
ECCENTRIC PULL-UP

If you cannot manage a full pull-up, use a block or partner to help you get into the raised position (elbows bent, head above the bar) and slowly lower. Working through the downward phase will strengthen the muscles and help to get you fit to do the full heave.

PTI Tip

When doing pull-ups, keep your body still and your movement controlled. Don't use momentum or swing actions to help you pull up to the bar.

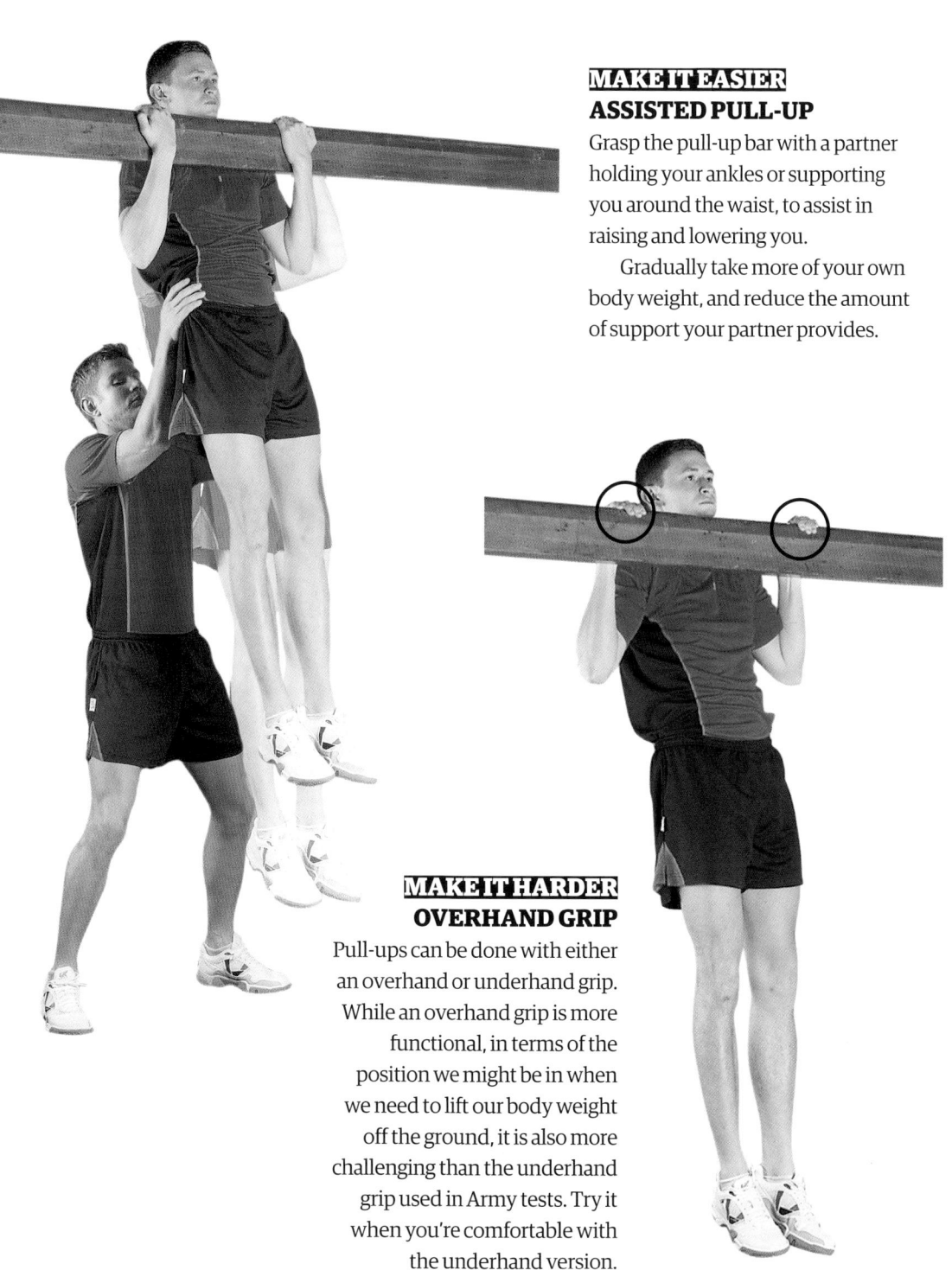

MAKE IT EASIER
ASSISTED PULL-UP

Grasp the pull-up bar with a partner holding your ankles or supporting you around the waist, to assist in raising and lowering you.

Gradually take more of your own body weight, and reduce the amount of support your partner provides.

MAKE IT HARDER
OVERHAND GRIP

Pull-ups can be done with either an overhand or underhand grip. While an overhand grip is more functional, in terms of the position we might be in when we need to lift our body weight off the ground, it is also more challenging than the underhand grip used in Army tests. Try it when you're comfortable with the underhand version.

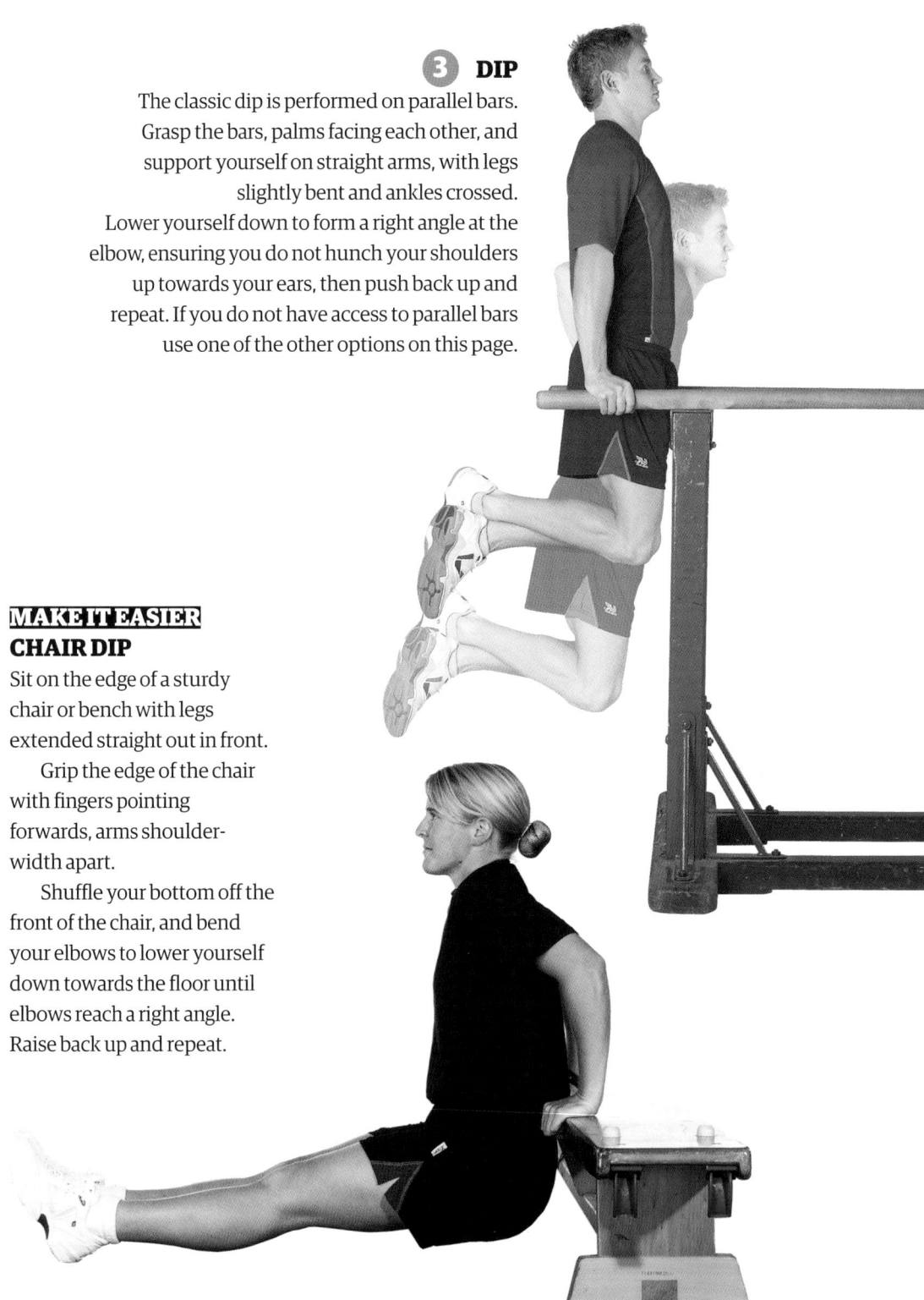

3 DIP

The classic dip is performed on parallel bars. Grasp the bars, palms facing each other, and support yourself on straight arms, with legs slightly bent and ankles crossed. Lower yourself down to form a right angle at the elbow, ensuring you do not hunch your shoulders up towards your ears, then push back up and repeat. If you do not have access to parallel bars use one of the other options on this page.

MAKE IT EASIER
CHAIR DIP

Sit on the edge of a sturdy chair or bench with legs extended straight out in front.

Grip the edge of the chair with fingers pointing forwards, arms shoulder-width apart.

Shuffle your bottom off the front of the chair, and bend your elbows to lower yourself down towards the floor until elbows reach a right angle. Raise back up and repeat.

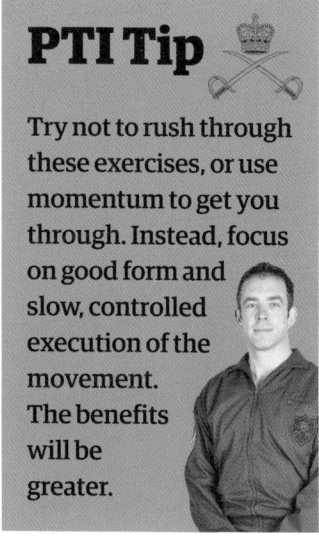

PTI Tip

Try not to rush through these exercises, or use momentum to get you through. Instead, focus on good form and slow, controlled execution of the movement. The benefits will be greater.

MAKE IT EASIER
KNEES-BENT CHAIR DIP

If you find the straight-leg dip too challenging, perform it with your knees bent. Gradually extend your legs out a little further as you get stronger.

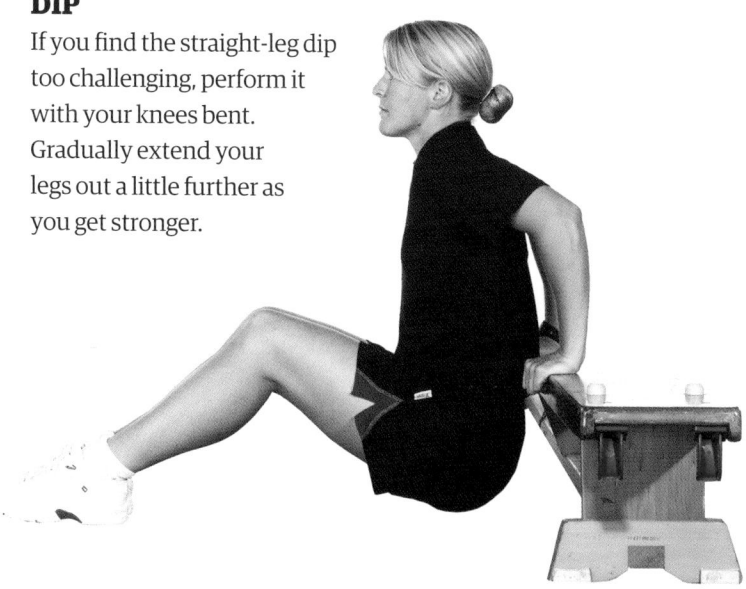

MAKE IT HARDER
DOUBLE CHAIR DIP

A more challenging version of the chair dip is to place your hands on one chair (or box) and put your feet on another chair opposite. Make sure both chairs are sturdy and placed on a stable surface.

Shuffle your bottom off the front of the chair and lower yourself down until elbows reach a right angle. Do not hunch your shoulders up to your ears.

You can progress this version further by adding weight to your lap, in the form of a Powerbag or medicine ball (pp.168-169).

Lower body exercises

4 STANDARD SQUAT

This compound exercise works the quads, glutes, hamstrings and calves.

Start with your feet hip-distance apart, toes turned slightly upwards and hands crossed over chest. Keeping your torso as upright as possible, bend the knees, leading with the bottom to lower towards the floor.

Do not bend further than a 90-degree angle at the knees. Pause in the lowered position, then raise and repeat.

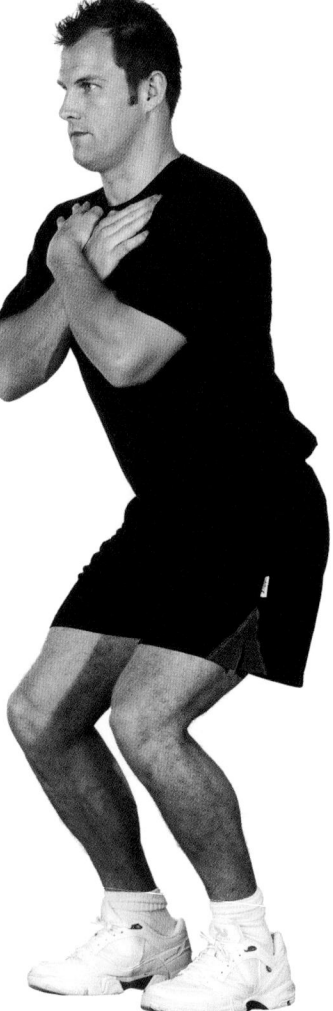

MAKE IT EASIER
QUARTER SQUAT
Use the same technique as for the standard squat, but bend only to 45 degrees rather than 90 degrees.

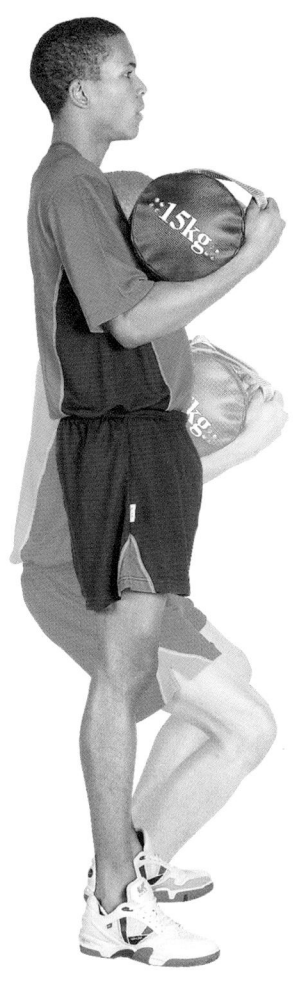

MAKE IT HARDER
SQUAT WITH POWERBAG

Start in the same stance as for the standard squat, but this time, instead of having your arms crossed over your chest, cradle a Powerbag, medicine ball or weight in front of you, close to your torso, to avoid putting excessive strain on your back. Now perform the squat as before.

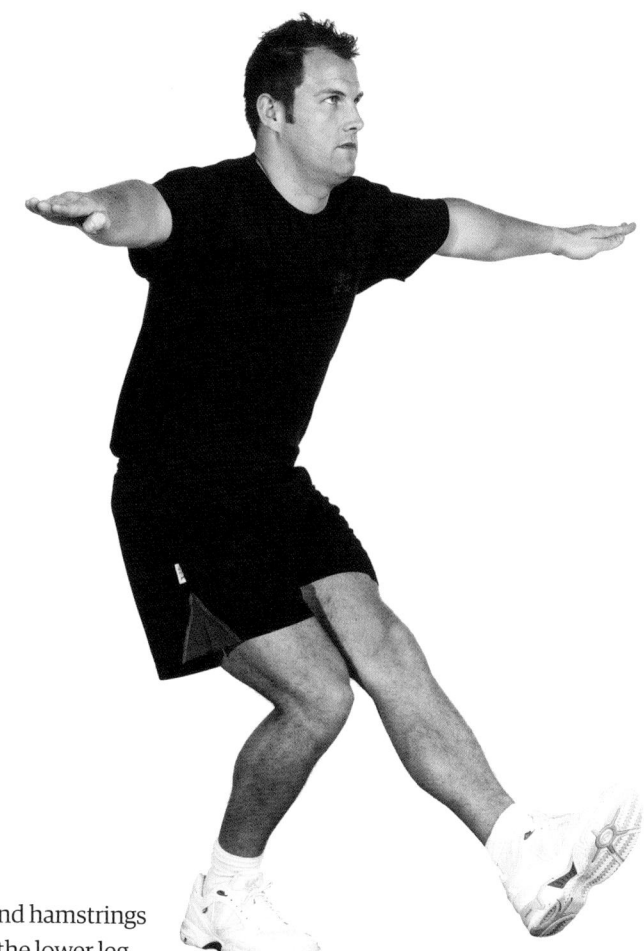

5 ONE-LEGGED SQUAT

This exercise works the quads, glutes and hamstrings as well as challenging the stabilisers in the lower leg. Take one foot off the floor and slightly bend the knee. Now bend the supporting leg, allowing the torso to tip forward as you lower, ensuring the knee stays in line with the foot, rather than rolling in or out. Lower as far as you comfortably can, then straighten and repeat. Swap sides.

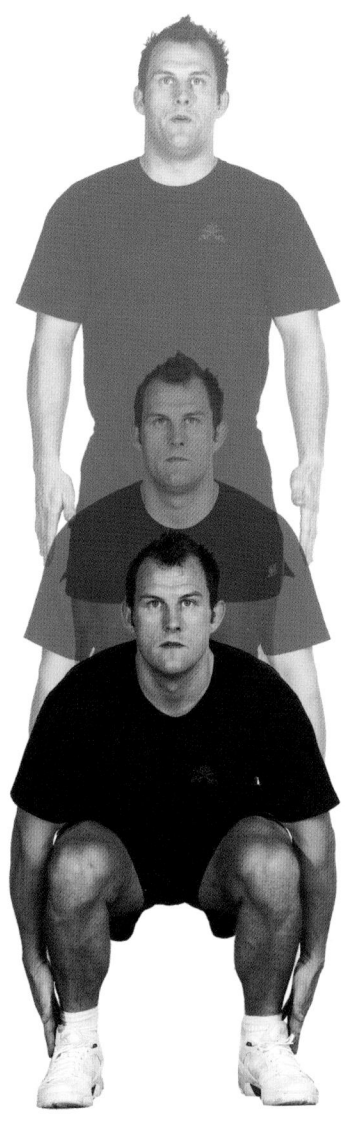

⑥ SQUAT JUMP

This advanced version of the squat adds speed and explosiveness, building power in the quads, glutes and hamstrings.

Stand with feet hip-distance apart and bend your knees until your hands touch the back of your ankles. From this position, leap up into the air, landing back down into the squat position, touching your ankles between each rep.

PTI Tip

Squats are a stock exercise for building leg strength – essential for Army tasks like marching and crossing obstacles, such as jumping to clear a ditch.

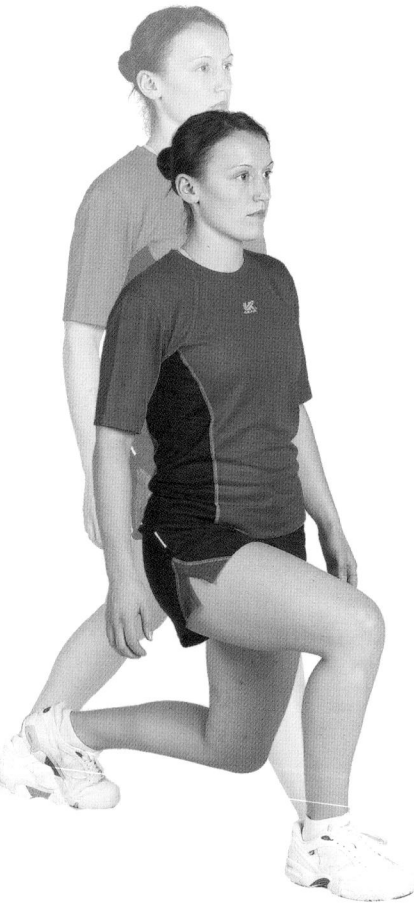

⑦ FORWARD LUNGE

This compound exercise works the quads, glutes and hamstrings. The inner thighs and hips (adductors and abductors) also work to balance and stabilise you.

Start with feet together and lunge forward, allowing the back knee to travel towards (but not touching) the floor and the front knee to bend, so that the knee is aligned above the ankle. Push back up through the front heel to the start position and repeat with the opposite leg. Holding dumbbells makes the exercise harder.

MAKE IT EASIER
BACKWARDS LUNGE

This version of the lunge puts less stress on the knees.

From a feet-together start position, lunge backwards with the right leg, allowing the right knee to travel towards the floor and the left knee to bend, so that it is above the left ankle. Push back up through the front heel to return to standing, and lunge back with the opposite leg.

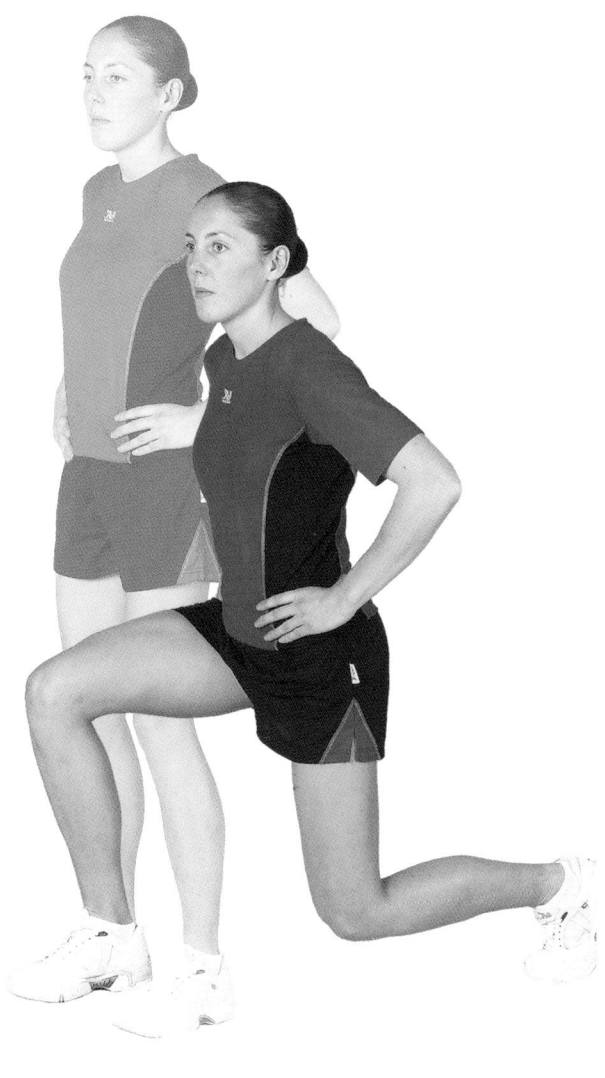

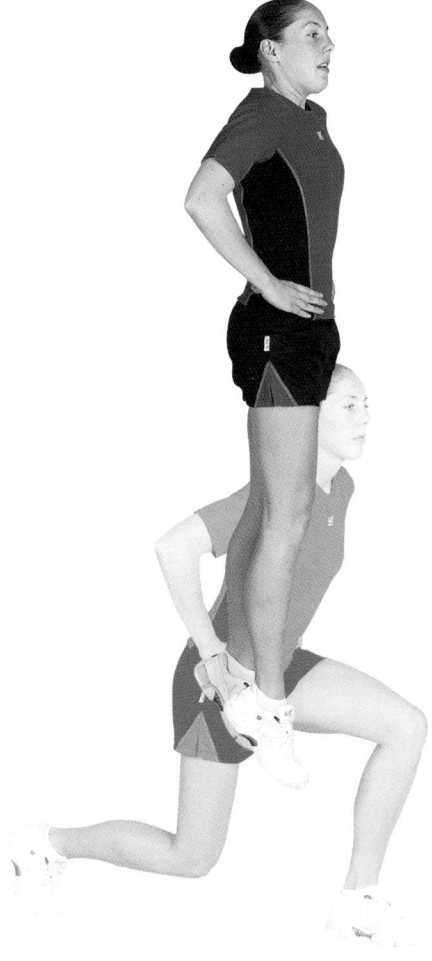

MAKE IT HARDER
LUNGE JUMP

This challenging exercise brings in speed, coordination and explosiveness. Start in a lunge position as in the stationary lunge, above. From here, leap up into the air, swapping feet midway, so that you land back in a lunge position on the other leg. Alternate from leg to leg to complete the set.

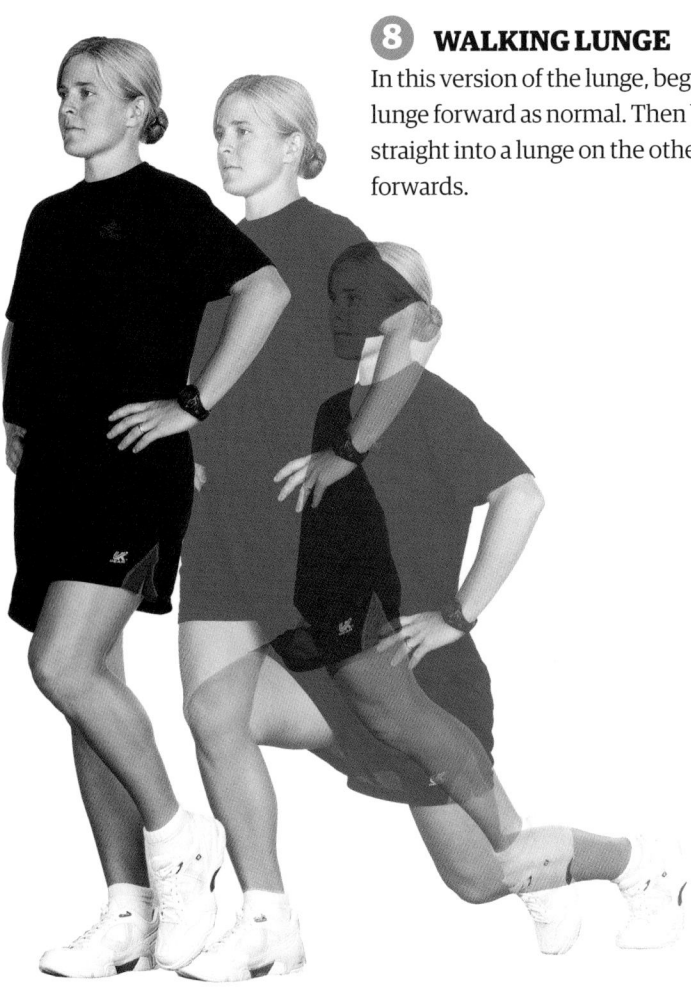

8 WALKING LUNGE

In this version of the lunge, begin with your feet together and lunge forward as normal. Then bring the back foot through to go straight into a lunge on the other leg. Continue to "walk" forwards.

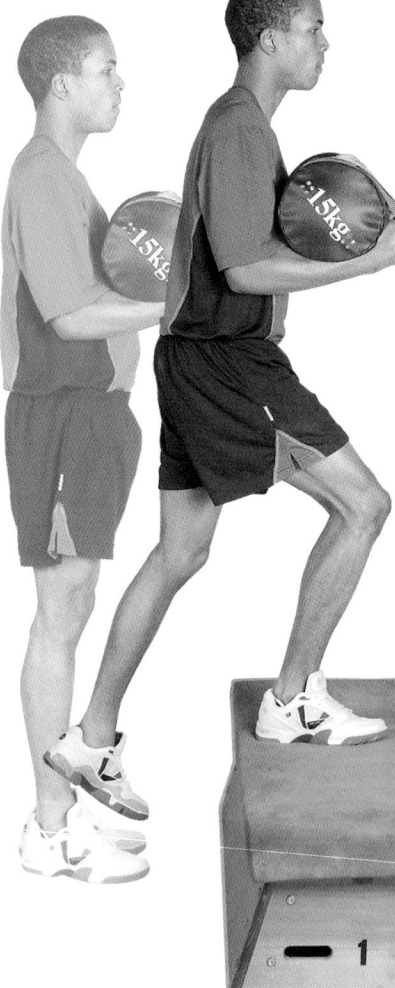

9 STEP-UP

Stand in front of a step (or stair) and step up on to the surface with your right foot, ensuring the whole foot makes contact with the platform. Immediately step up with the left foot, so both feet are on the platform, then step back down with the right, and left foot. Go straight into the next repetition, stepping up with the left foot. Ensure you do not bend from the waist as you step up. To make the exercise harder, hold a weight in each hand, keeping arms straight and by your sides.

MAKE IT HARDER
STEP-UP WITH KNEE RAISE

Stand in front of a step with your feet together.

Step up with your right foot and drive through with your left leg, bringing this left knee up to your chest before placing first the left and then the right foot back on to the floor.

Swap to lead with your left leg, and alternate between the two legs to complete the set.

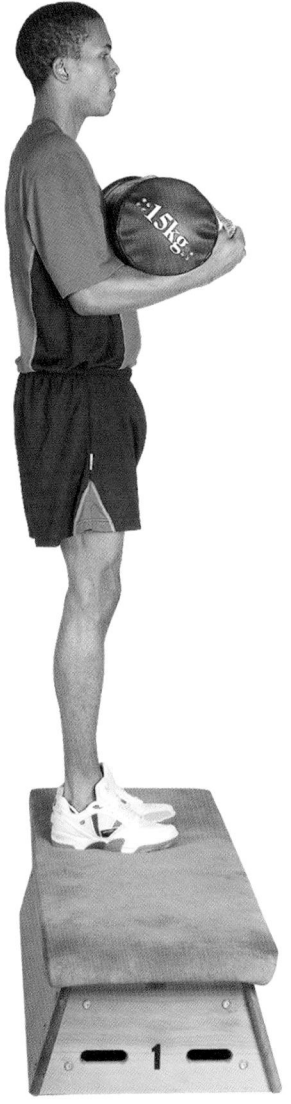

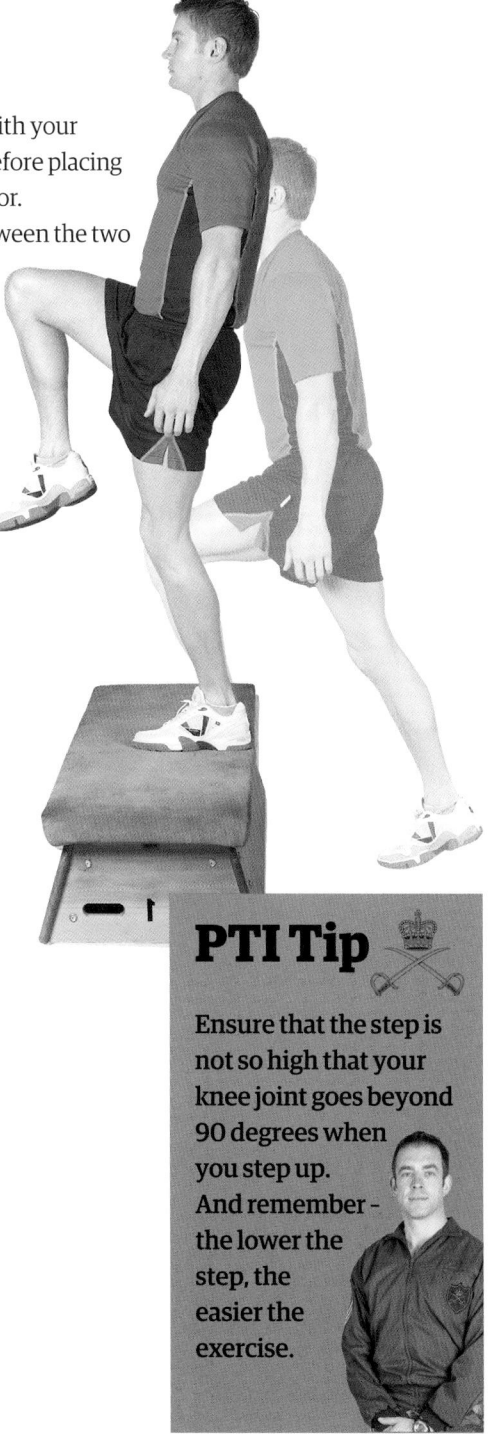

PTI Tip

Ensure that the step is not so high that your knee joint goes beyond 90 degrees when you step up. And remember – the lower the step, the easier the exercise.

Strong to the core

You may have heard the term "core stability". This refers to a specific type of training which focuses on the deep-set trunk muscles and aims to enhance these muscles' ability to stabilise the spine and pelvis. A well-functioning core provides a stable base from which to move your limbs with maximum efficiency and power, and with minimal risk of injury. The primary role of these "stabiliser" muscles is to hold the body - or part of it - stable, sometimes while another part of the body is moving.

For example, the core stabilisers are recruited to hold the spine in its usual S-shape, before you pick a weight up off the floor. While the core muscles do not need brute strength, they do need to be able to "switch on" when they are needed, and to be able to work continuously, at a low level of contraction.

That is why core exercises often don't involve lifting weights – in fact some don't even involve moving at all. But don't make the mistake of thinking that the core stabilisers only work during specific core stability exercises. These muscles are active in almost every movement we make, so to a certain extent they are being trained all the time, but the focus on proper technique and good posture during dedicated core stability work helps to target them more closely.

PTI Tip

Drawing your belly button towards your spine helps engage the core stabilisers. Try to get into the habit of engaging the core before you perform any exercise (not just by sucking in your stomach and holding your breath) to protect the spine and work these important muscles.

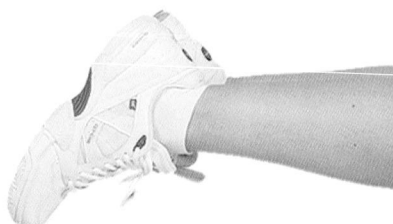

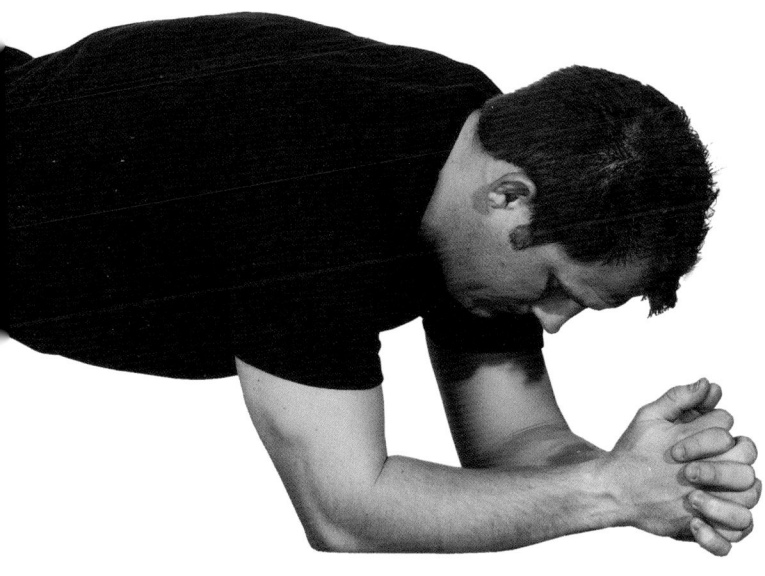

Abs and back exercises

10 PLANK

Lie face down on a mat, with elbows below shoulders and forearms pointing forwards. Draw your belly button towards your spine and raise your body off the floor, so that your weight is resting on your forearms and toes, and forms a perfect straight line. Do not let your back sag in the middle. Hold for the required length of time, breathing freely.

MAKE IT EASIER
MODIFIED PLANK

If you are not able to hold the full plank position for even a few seconds, try this modified version, and work your way up to the full plank.

Begin as before, but this time, when you raise your body on to your elbows, keep the knees on the floor, so that your body forms a straight line from your knees to the top of your head.

MAKE IT HARDER

If the full plank feels easy, try extending alternate legs up into the air while still in position, keeping the body stable and not rocking from side to side.

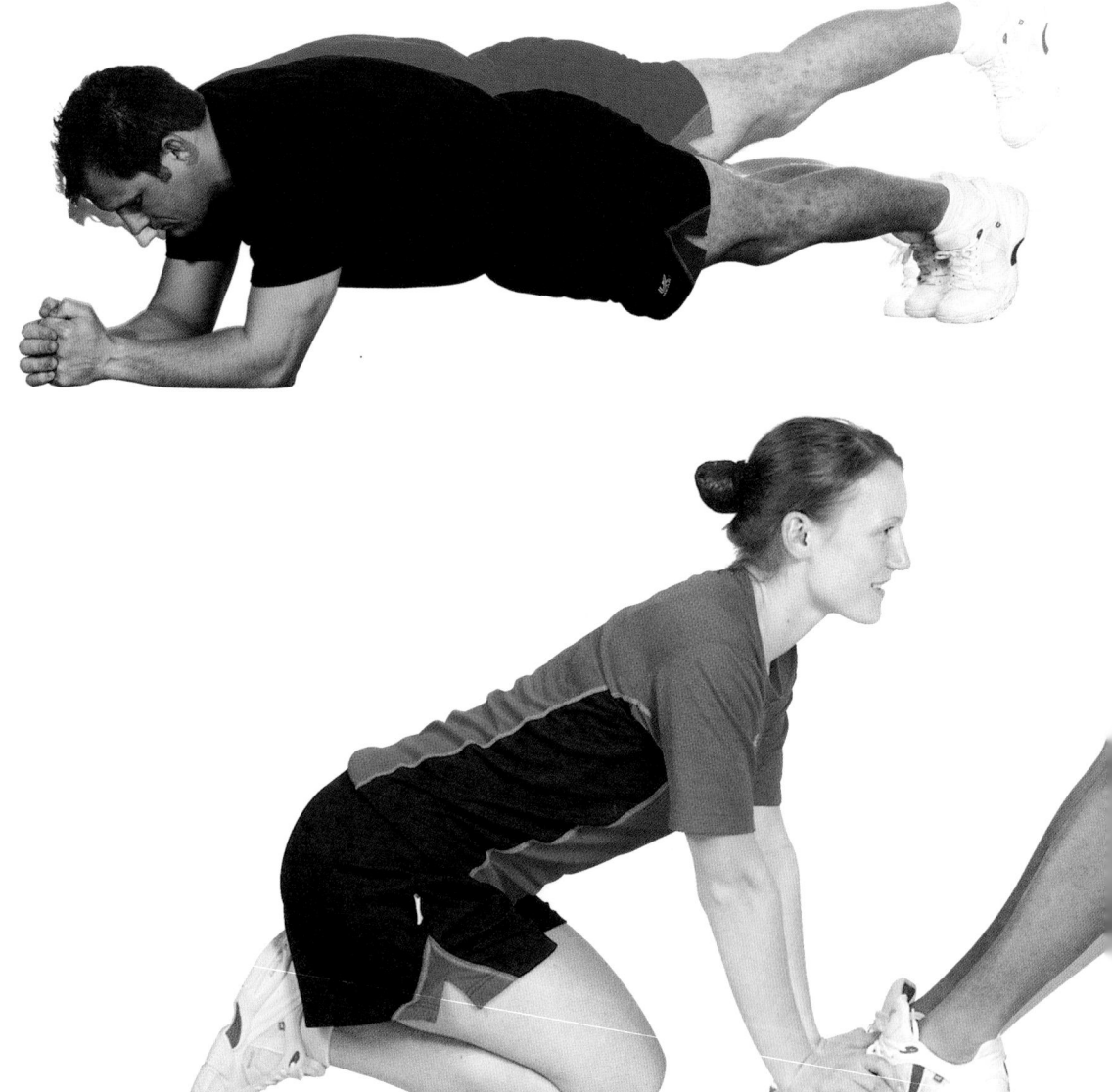

11 SIDE PLANK

This position works the transversus abdominis, quadratus lumborum and obliques.

Lie on your side, propped up on the lower elbow, with your body in a straight line. Raise your body up, so that your weight is resting on your elbow and the lower foot. You can keep the upper arm close to the body, or raise it up straight in the air (a balance challenge).

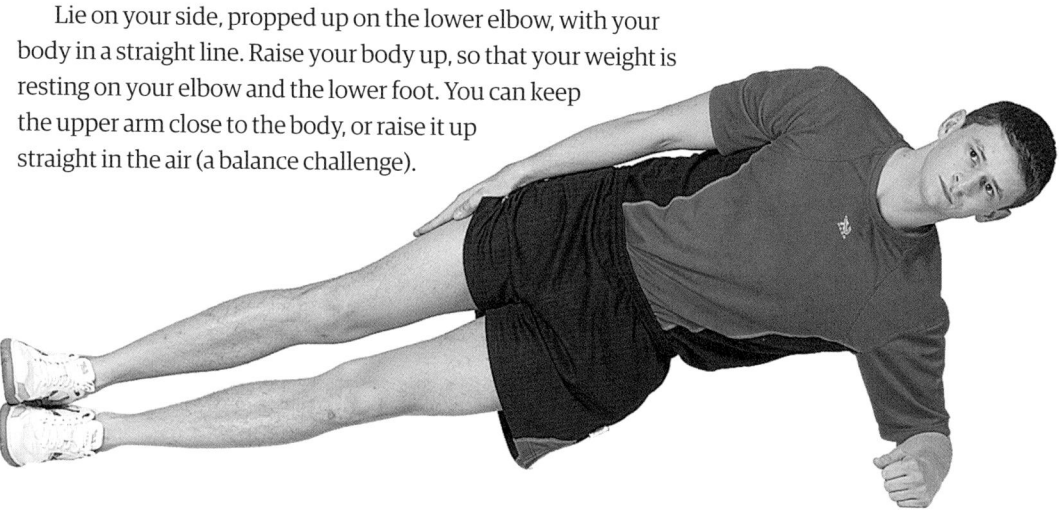

12 SIT-UP

This is the classic exercise for strengthening the rectus abdominis ("six-pack"). It also works the external obliques and hip flexors.

In the Army's two-minute sit-up test (p.115),the exercise is performed with your feet anchored by a partner or low object. This position introduces the hip flexors, so is less taxing on the abdominals.

Start by lying on the floor with your knees bent and feet anchored. Have your hands across your chest with your fingers touching each collarbone and your elbows tucked in.

Maintaining a flat back, curl your head, shoulders and torso off the floor until your torso is in an upright position, then roll back down through the spine to the start position and repeat.

MAKE IT EASIER
HALF-SIT

If you find the full sit-up too difficult, start off with this easier version, which works the rectus abdominis and external obliques.

Lie on the floor with knees slightly bent. Place your hands on your thighs and curl up, sliding your hands up along your legs until your fingers extend beyond your knees. Lower and repeat.

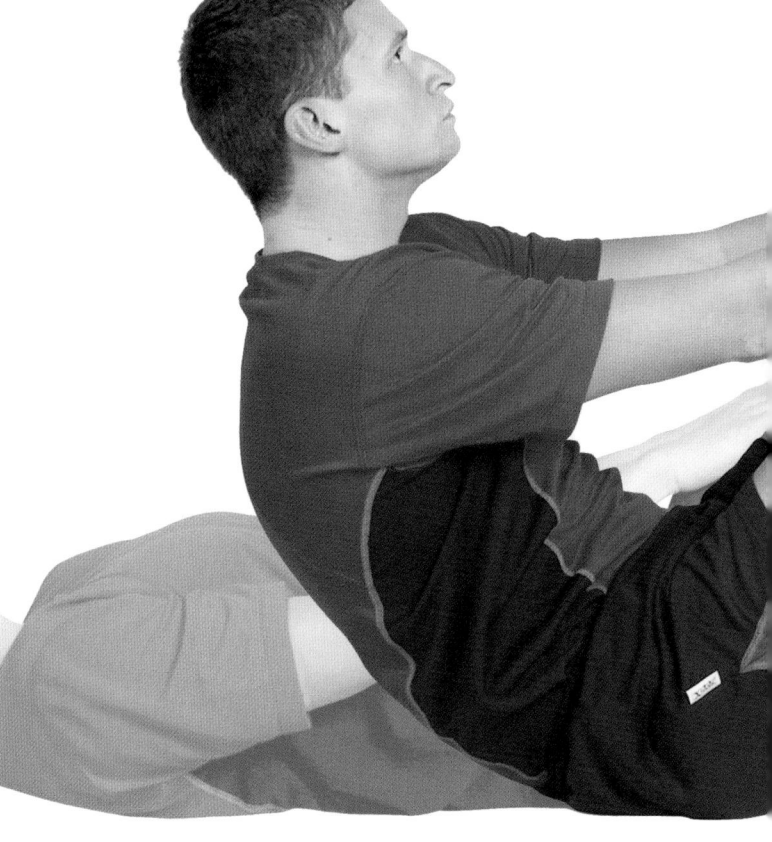

MAKE IT HARDER
CRUNCH

This advanced variation of a sit-up works most of the core muscles, as well as the hip flexors.

Start lying on the floor with your hands beside your head. Sit up, bringing your knees to your chest, and then rock back, fully extending your legs before bringing the knees in to meet the chest again. Do not allow the feet to touch the floor in between reps.

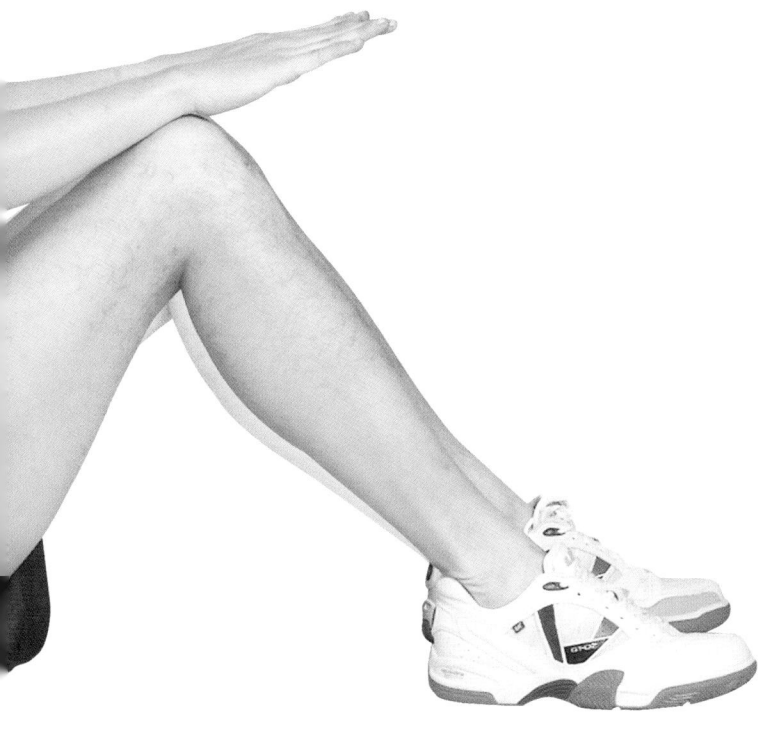

⑬ TWIST SIT-UP

The element of rotation in this sit-up focuses on the external obliques. Begin by lying on the floor with hands beside your head and knees slightly bent, feet on the floor. Curl your torso off the floor, rotating it to the right as you simultaneously bring your right knee in towards your chest.

Lower, taking the foot back to the floor, then curl up, twisting to the left and bringing the left knee into the chest. Continue to alternate from side to side for the set.

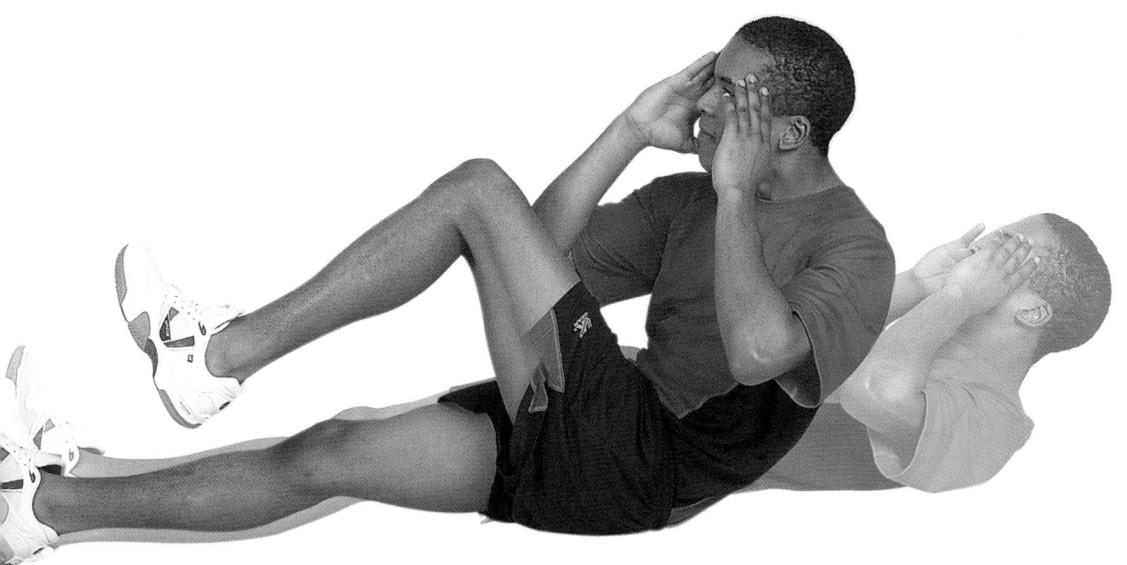

14 **DORSAL RAISE**

Lie face down on the floor with fingertips clasped in front of your chin. Lift your torso off the floor, being careful not to jerk or force the movement, and keeping your head in line with the spine.

Pause and lower to repeat.

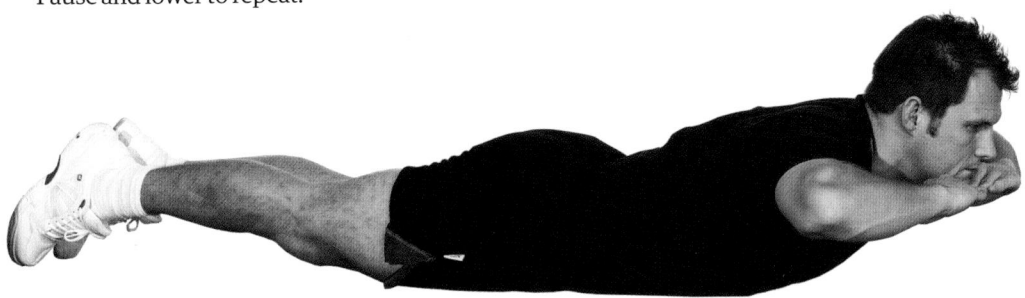

MAKE IT HARDER

SUPERMANS

A good progression from, or alternative to, dorsal raises, Supermans also work the back extensor muscles.

Lie face down on the floor, with arms extended flat on the floor overhead. Lift your right arm and left leg off the floor simultaneously, keeping the hips and pelvis centred, and your head in line with the spine. Lower, and then lift your left arm and right leg off the floor.

Continue to alternate for the set.

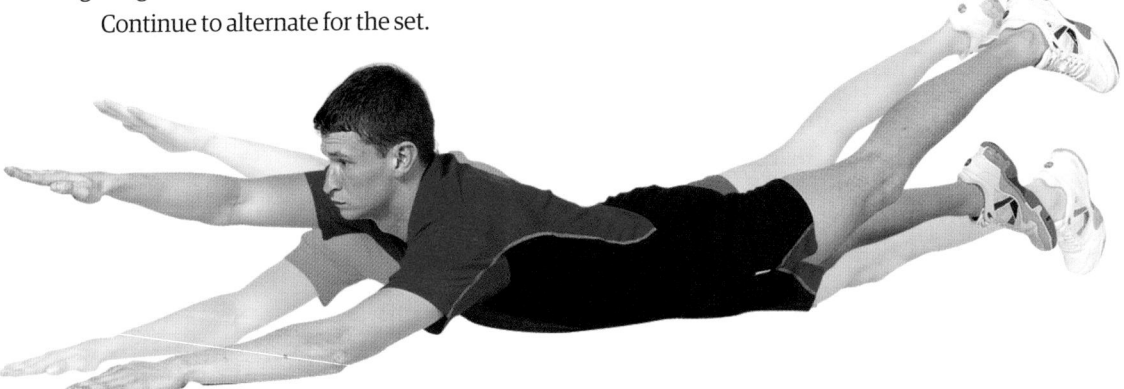

BRIDGE

This exercise strengthens the lower back extensors, the glutes and the inner thigh muscles.

Lie on the floor with knees bent and feet flat. Raise the body up to form a straight line between knees and shoulders and hold for the required length of time (see programmes pp.124–147).

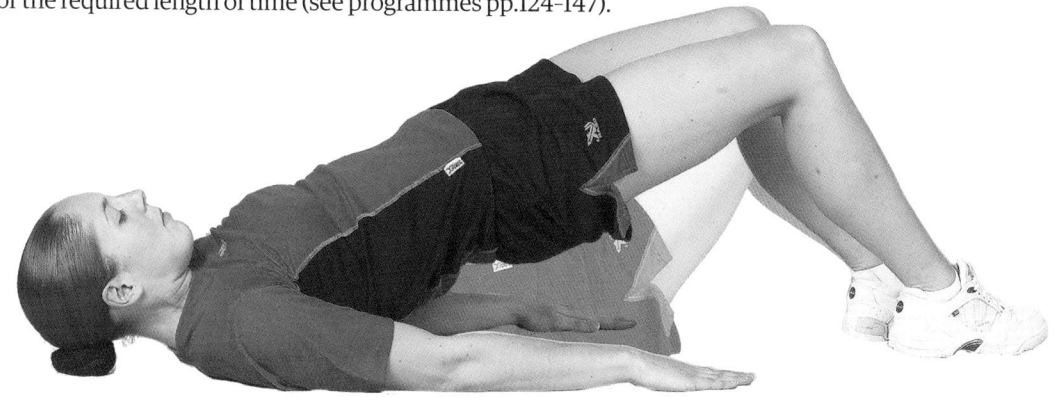

MAKE IT HARDER
BRIDGE WITH LEG EXTENSION

Once you can do the bridge comfortably, do the same as above, but once your pelvis is raised, alternately extend one leg and then the other, without allowing the pelvis to rock from side to side.

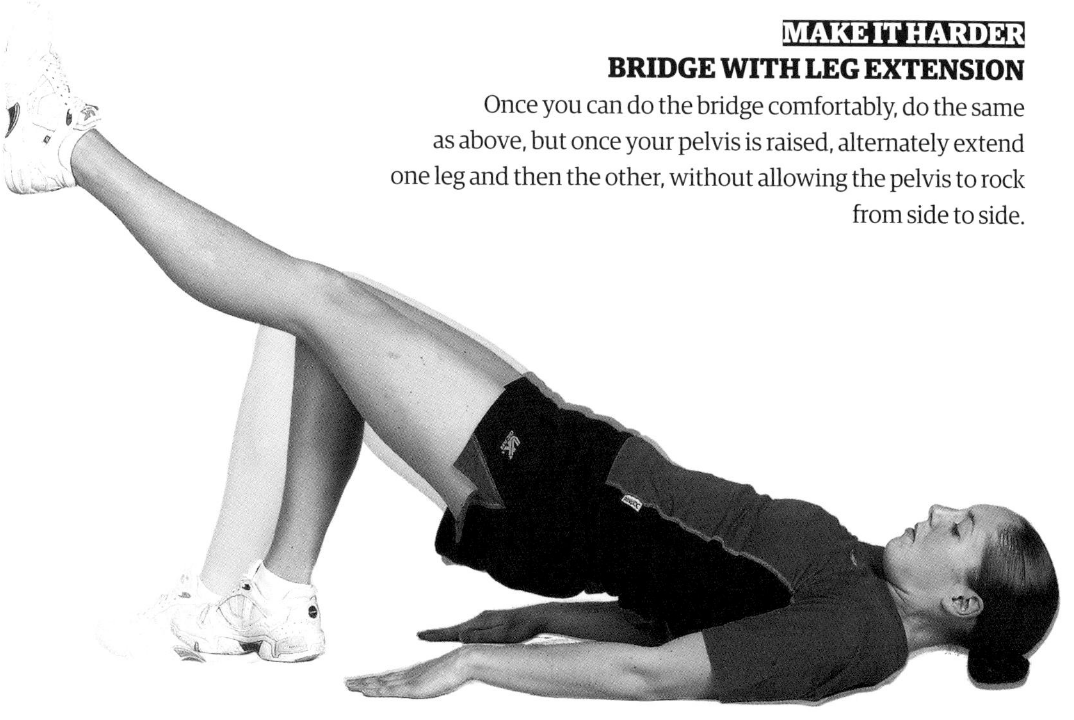

Additional exercises

You can add or substitute the exercises that follow for those in the 12-week Army Fitness Programmes (pp.124-147), to give more variety and to hone in on specific areas, enabling you to keep challenging yourself as you get stronger.

More upper body exercises

BENCH PRESS WITH DUMBBELLS

This is a good alternative to press-ups, working the chest, shoulders and triceps.

Lie on a bench or step with a dumbbell in each hand, resting just above your chest (below). Extend the arms upwards, keeping them level with your breastbone, in an arc-like motion until your arms are fully outstretched. Pause, then lower and repeat.

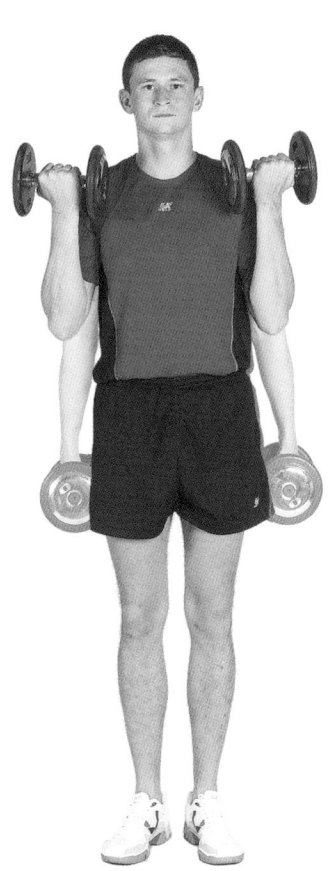

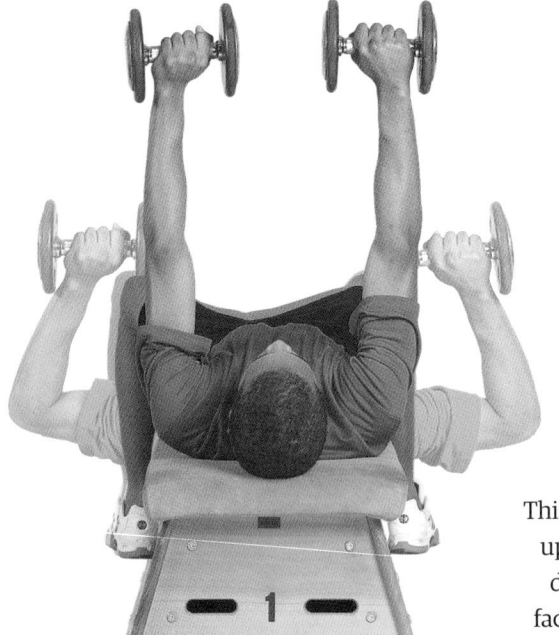

BICEPS CURL WITH DUMBBELLS

This exercise targets the biceps on the front of the upper arm used in pull-ups. Stand with feet hip-distance apart, a dumbbell in each hand, palms facing your thighs. Bend your elbows to raise the weights up, allowing the arm to rotate so that when the weights reach the front of your shoulders, the palms are facing you. Pause, then lower and repeat.

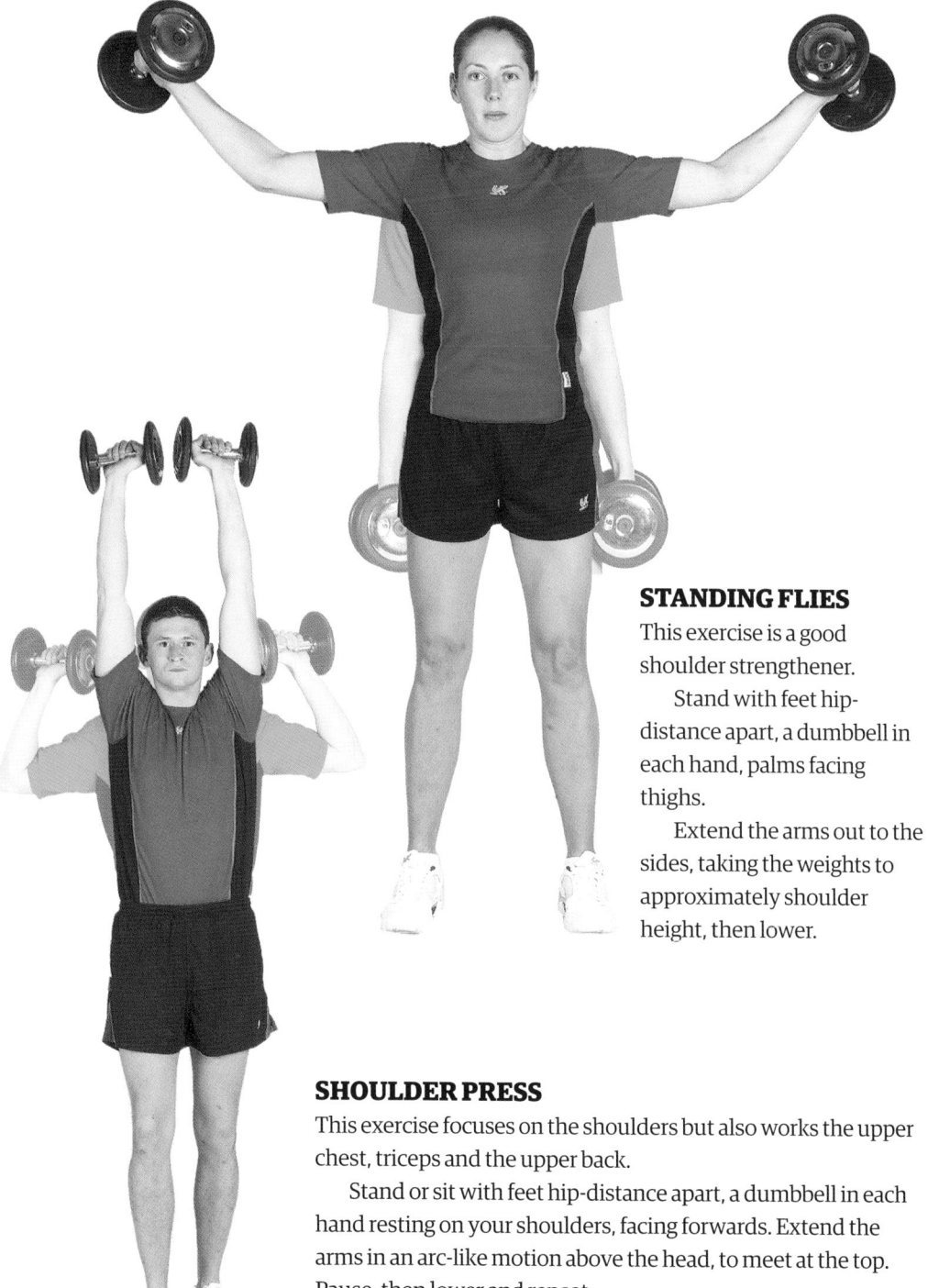

STANDING FLIES

This exercise is a good shoulder strengthener.

Stand with feet hip-distance apart, a dumbbell in each hand, palms facing thighs.

Extend the arms out to the sides, taking the weights to approximately shoulder height, then lower.

SHOULDER PRESS

This exercise focuses on the shoulders but also works the upper chest, triceps and the upper back.

Stand or sit with feet hip-distance apart, a dumbbell in each hand resting on your shoulders, facing forwards. Extend the arms in an arc-like motion above the head, to meet at the top. Pause, then lower and repeat.

SINGLE-ARM ROW

This is a good alternative to the pull-up if you don't have the right equipment. It mimics the underhand grip most closely.

Kneel side-on to a bench, with a dumbbell in the hand furthest from the bench. Have your back straight, stomach pulled in and neck in line with the spine. Start with the arm relaxed, hanging straight down holding the dumbbell. Then, keeping the back still, bend the arm at the elbow to bring the weight up to the front of the shoulder. Pause, lower and repeat. Swap sides between sets.

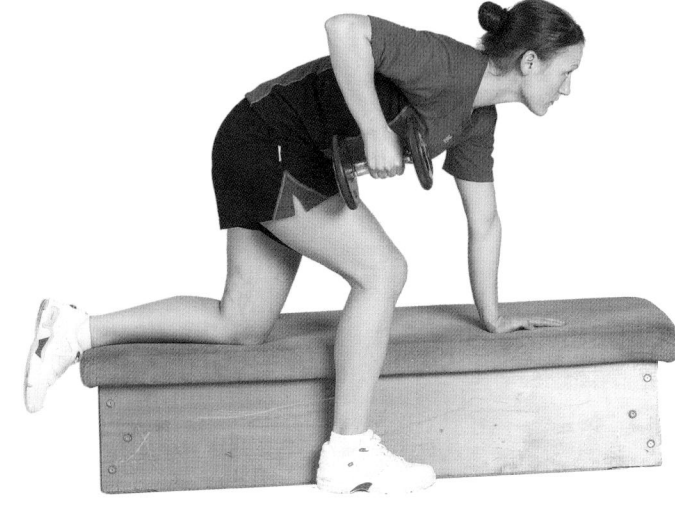

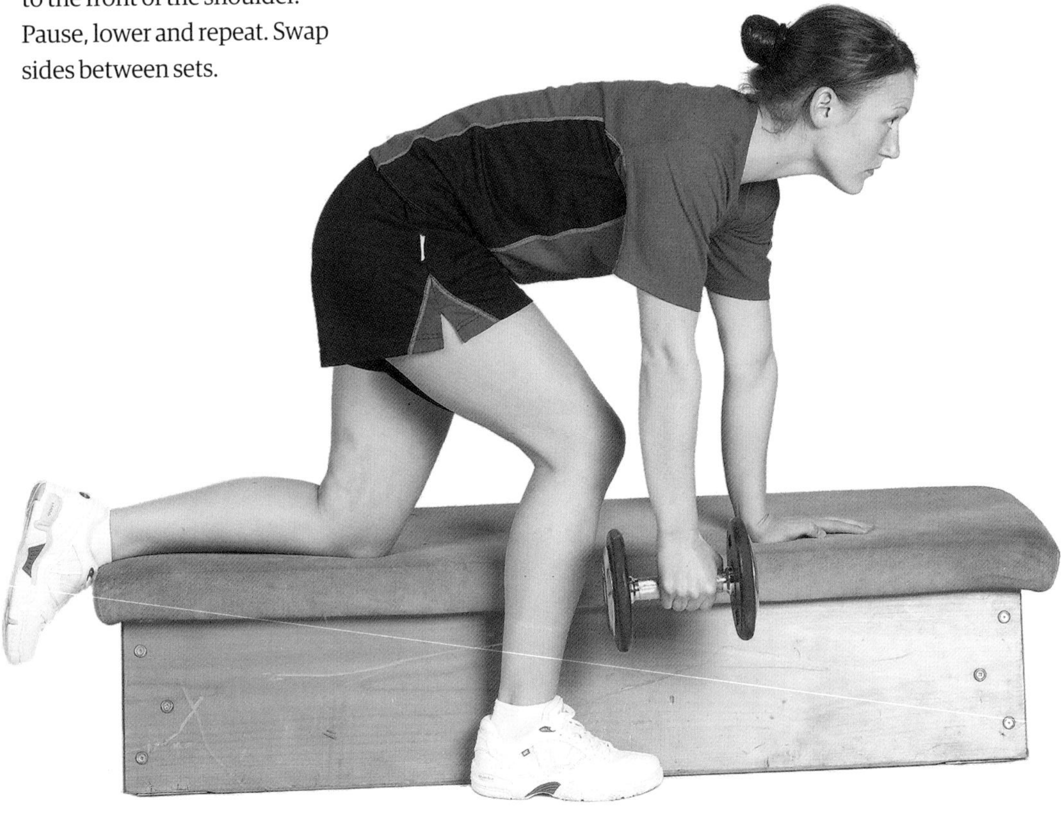

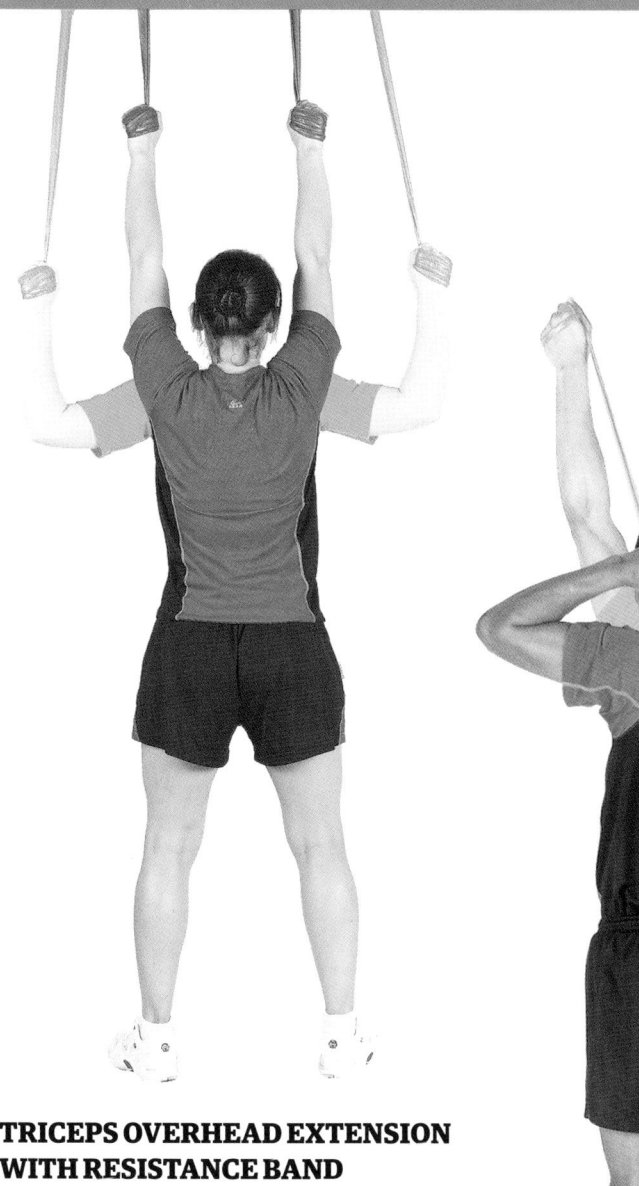

LAT PULL-DOWN WITH RESISTANCE BAND

This exercise (left) is another good alternative to a pull-up and uses the same muscle groups as an overhand grip.

Hook the resistance band over a rail or bar (or use a door attachment, see p.169). Take an end of the resistance band in each hand and stand or sit with palms facing forwards, arms extended. Now bend the arms, squeezing the shoulder blades together, to bring the handles of the resistance band towards your shoulders. Pause, then extend the arms again and repeat.

TRICEPS OVERHEAD EXTENSION WITH RESISTANCE BAND

You can do this triceps-strengthening exercise (right) either using a resistance band or holding a dumbbell. It is a good alternative to the dip.

Take one end of the resistance band in your left hand and stand on the other end of it with your right foot. Take your arm up beside your head and bend the arm at the elbow behind you until your arm is straight, adjusting the resistance until there is some tension in the band.

Now extend the arm overhead, resisting the band, until your elbow is straight. Pause, then lower and repeat. Swap sides between sets.

More lower body exercises

CALF RAISE

This exercise hones in on the calf muscles at the back of the lower legs. It is a great exercise for people who have suffered from Achilles tendon problems . If that's you, focus on the lowering phase rather than the rising phase.

Stand on the edge of a step or stair, with your heels off the end. (You may need to hold on to a support.) Raise up on to the toes, as high as you can, and then lower the heels down below the level of the step. Raise up from here and repeat.

BASIC BURPEE

Burpees are the ultimate in compound training, because they use a whole range of muscles, not just in the legs but in the trunk and upper body, too.

Stand with feet shoulder-width apart. Bend your knees and lower body towards the floor. Once your hands touch the floor, thrust your legs to the rear into a press-up position, keeping back straight and stomach pulled in. Then bring your knees back in, take the weight off your hands and stand up.

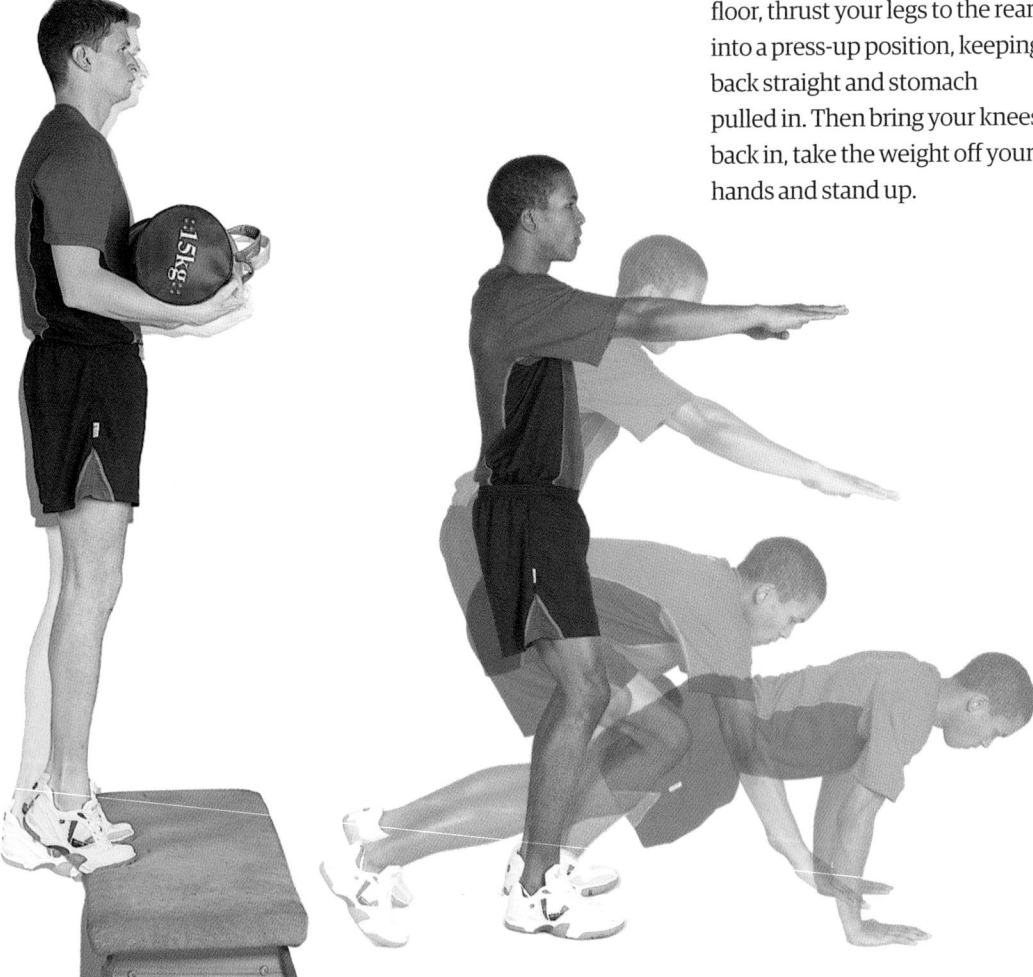

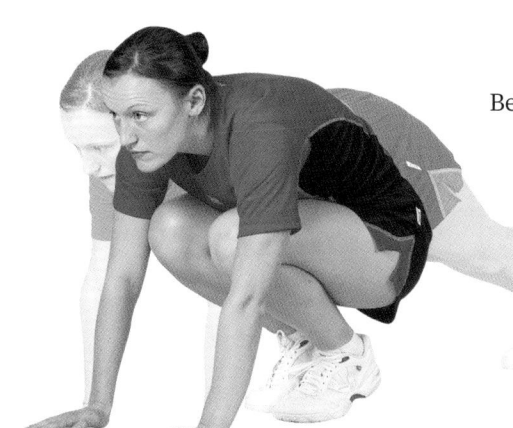

SQUAT THRUST

Begin with your body in a "plank" position, with arms straight and under your shoulders, legs extended, and weight on toes. Jump to bring the feet in towards the chest, and then extend them out straight again. Keep your back straight and abs contracted.

SQUAT THRUST WITH SINGLE LEGS

If you find the full squat thrust exercise too difficult, this single-leg version is an easier alternative. Start in the same position as above, but bring only one leg into the chest at a time, so that you are springing forward on one leg as you extend the other one out to the back.

To make squat thrusts even easier, you can perform them with your hands on a raised surface instead of the floor.

BURPEE WITH PRESS-UP AND JUMP

In this more challenging version, perform the burpee as opposite, but when you are in the press-up position, bend your elbows and actually perform a press-up. Then bring your knees back in and from this squat position, explode upwards into a jump to standing.

SUPINE HAMSTRING CURL

This exercise strengthens the hamstrings, as well as improving muscular endurance in the lower back.

Lie face up with your feet on a Swiss ball and arms beside you on the floor. Lift your hips up, so that your body forms a straight line from feet to head. Now, bending your knees, draw the ball in towards your bottom using your feet.

Keep the hips raised, then extend the legs out again.

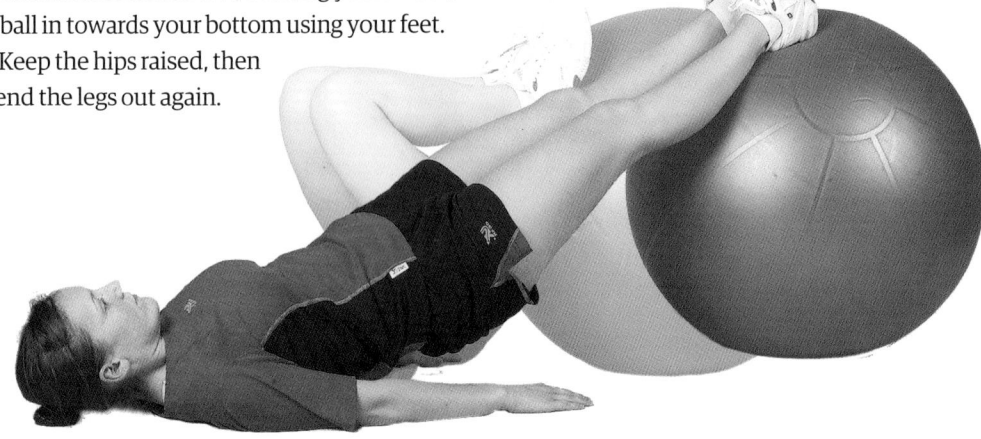

STANDING LEG CROSSOVER

This exercise works the muscles along the inner thigh, the adductors.

Tie one end of a resistance band around something sturdy, and loop the other end around your right ankle. Move away from the attachment point until there is sufficient tension in the band and your right leg is lifted out to the side. Now bring your right leg in, allowing it to cross over in front of the left leg. Keep toes facing forward. Return to start position and repeat.

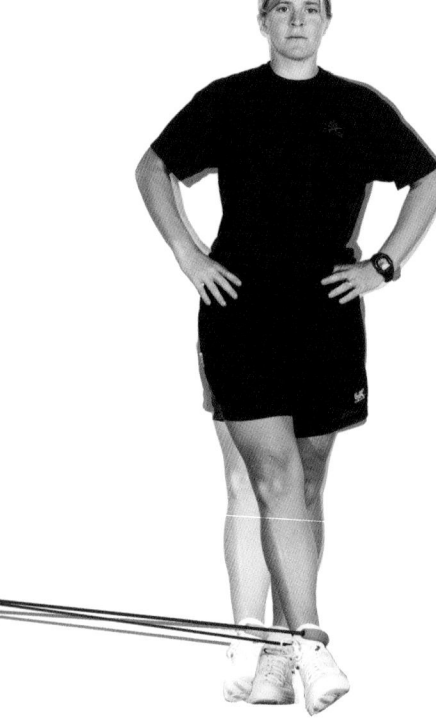

STANDING LEG RAISE

This exercise works the muscles along the outer thigh and hip, the abductors.

Leaving the resistance band in the same place as in the crossover exercise (opposite), face the opposite way and secure the free end around your right ankle (the one furthest from the resistance band). Move away from the attachment point until there is some tension in the band. Now lift your right leg directly out to the side, working against the resistance of the band. Lower and repeat. Swap sides.

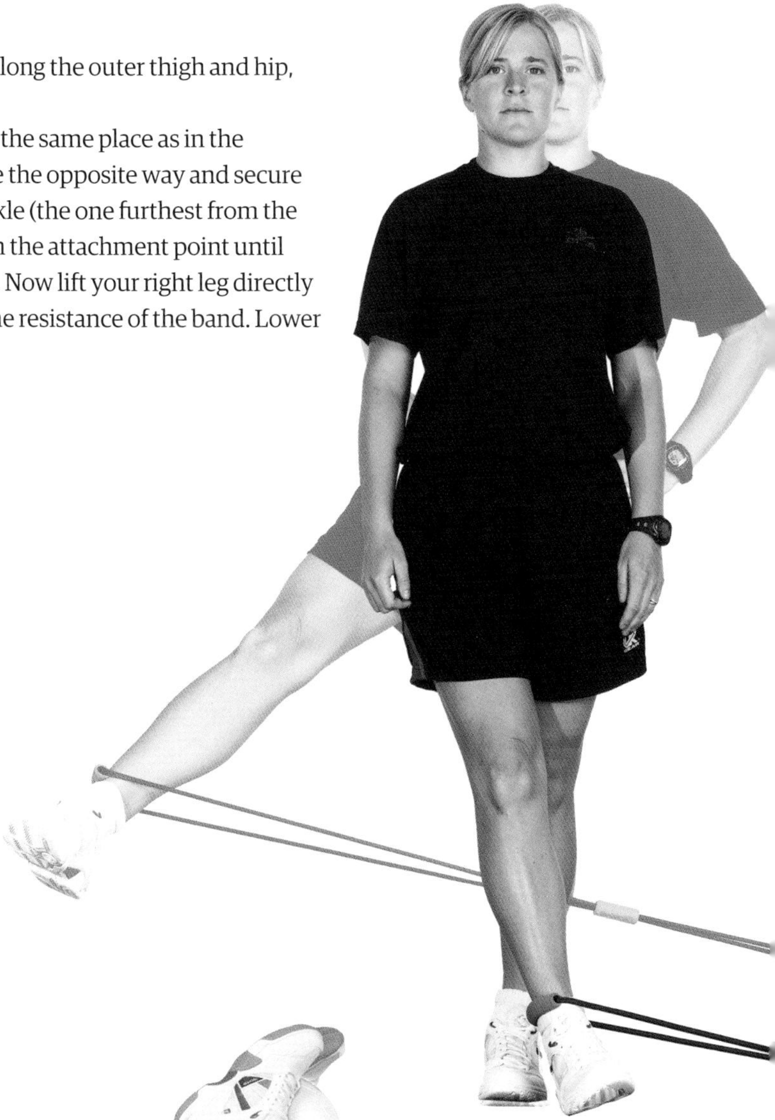

PRONE HAMSTRING CURL

Another great exercise for honing in on the hamstrings.

Place a medicine ball or other weight between your feet and lie prone on the floor. Pick the ball up between your feet and bend your knees, drawing the ball in towards your bottom. Pause, then straighten the legs to lower the ball and repeat.

You can also do this exercise with a resistance band: tie both ends securely to a stable surface close to your feet and loop it around your ankles, so that when you bend your legs you are working against the elastic resistance.

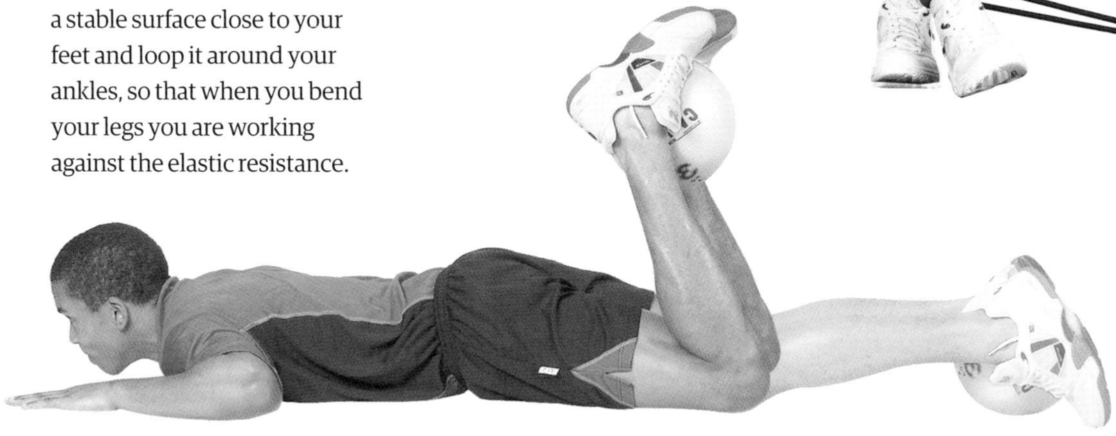

More abs and back exercises

SEATED LEG EXTENSION

Another challenging sit-up variation, mainly working the rectus abdominis ("six-pack") and hip flexors.

Sit on a chair or bench, with your hands supporting you on the back edge or sides. Start with knees bent into chest, then extend the legs out in front, allowing the torso to move slightly back as you do so. Pause, then draw the legs back in.

SUPINE PLANK

This plank position works the stabilisers in the back, as well as the glutes and the muscles between the shoulder blades.

Start face up on your mat, propped up on your elbows and legs extended. Now lift your body off the floor to form a straight line. Keep your neck in line with the spine by looking at the ceiling.

LATERAL FLEXION

Lateral flexion (bending to the side) works both sets of obliques and the muscles that flex the spine to the side.

Hold a dumbbell or weight in one hand by your side and stand with feet hip-distance apart. Keeping the hips centred, bend directly to the side as far as you comfortably can.

Come back to the centre and bend to the opposite side. Repeat, holding the weight in the other hand. Continue to alternate for the set.

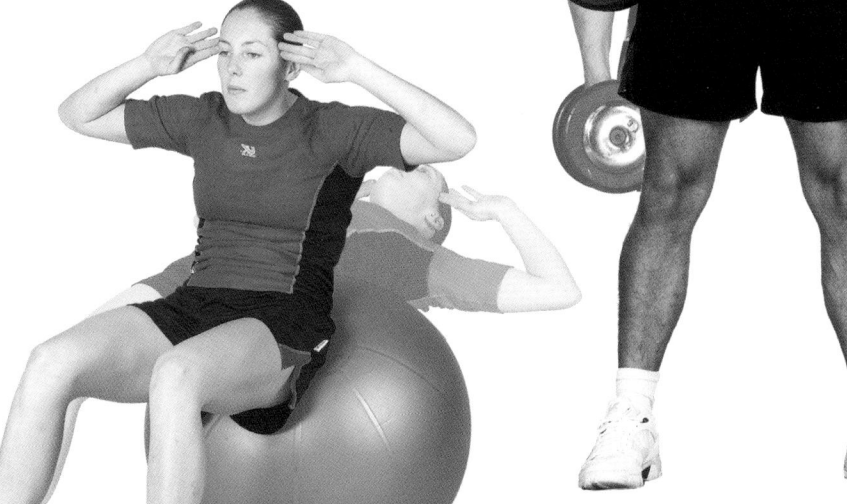

SWISS BALL SIT-UP

Lie on a Swiss ball with your feet on the floor. Adjust yourself so that your bottom is just off the front of the ball, with buttocks unclenched and your hands either beside your head or crossed over your chest.

Contracting the abdominals, raise and flex the upper torso as far as you can without moving the ball underneath you. Pause, then lower and repeat.

BACK EXTENSION ON BALL

This is an excellent exercise for the back extensors, because it allows the back to come from a flexed position to an extended one, working through a greater range than is possible on the floor.

Lie face down on a Swiss ball with your feet anchored against the join of the wall and the floor, or get a friend to hold your feet. Adjust your position until your torso is lower than your hips, and put your hands beside your head.

Now raise the torso up until it is just a bit further than in a straight line with the legs, using the back and bottom muscles. Hold, then lower and repeat.

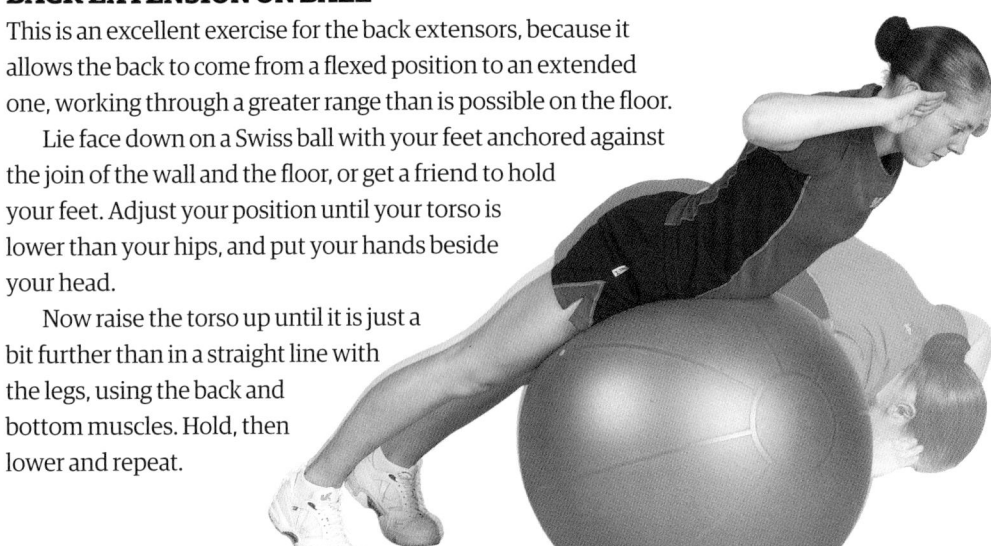

PIKE ON SWISS BALL

This advanced exercise works the core stabilisers, the rectus abdominis, hip flexors and many upper body muscles, too.

Lie face down over a Swiss ball and shunt forwards until only your shins are on the ball and your weight is supported on your hands, arms shoulder-width apart.

Contract the abdominals and tilt the pelvis so your back is in a straight line with the legs.

Now draw the ball in towards your torso by contracting the abs and lifting your hips into the air. Keep your shoulders drawn back and don't arch the back.

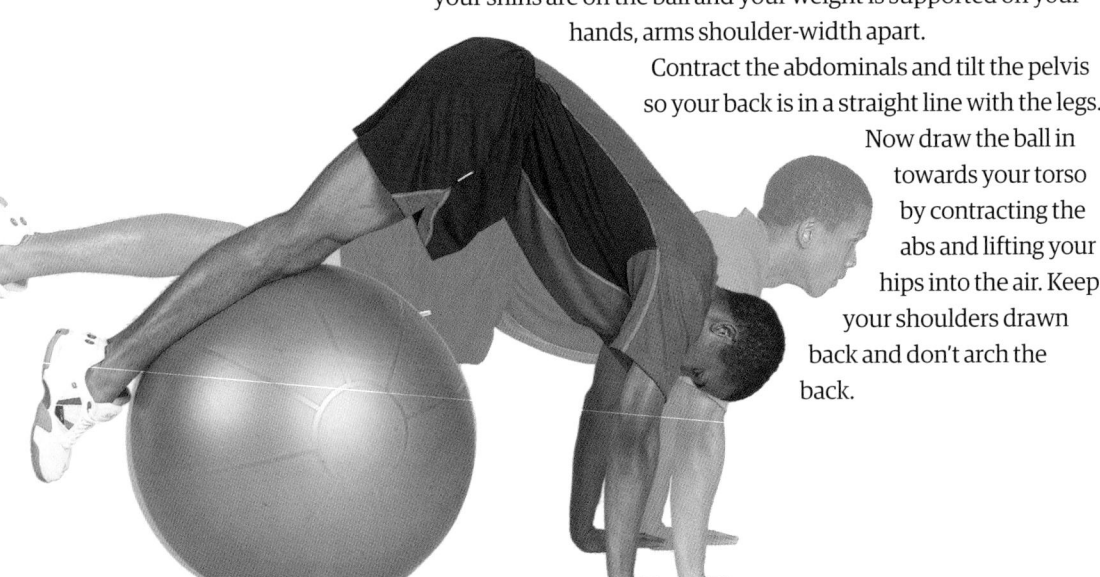

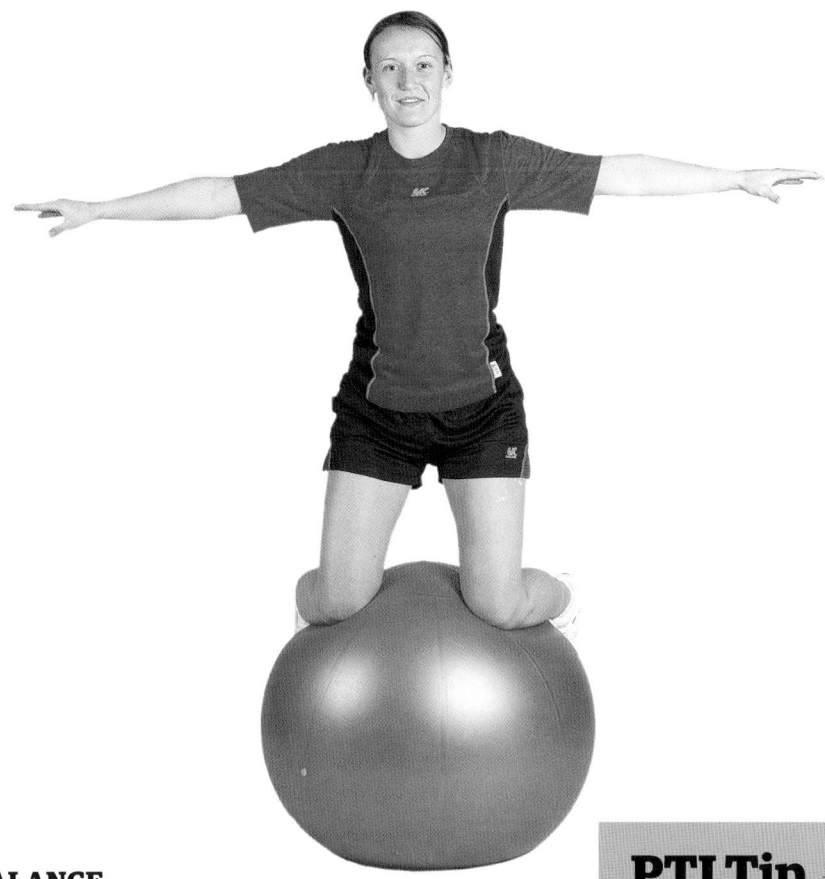

BALL BALANCE

This is an advanced exercise to challenge your balance and get all your core stabilisers firing.

Stand in front of a Swiss ball. If you are new to this exercise, either get a friend to stand on the opposite side of the ball to help you balance, or have a wall on the other side of the ball, which you can hold on to if necessary.

In a swift movement, put your hands on the ball and rock your body forward to place both knees simultaneously on the ball. Then roll the pelvis forward so that you are in a kneeling-up position and take your hands away.

You need to constantly adjust your body position to stay balanced – really focus on using the core muscles to help you.

Hold the pose for as long as you can without falling off.

PTI Tip

When the ball balance is easy, you can add extra challenges, such as getting someone to throw you a ball while you balance, making tiny figures of eight with the ball, or balancing with your eyes shut.

Four-week strength start-up programme

If you've rarely set foot in a gym, or feel you lack muscular strength, this start-up programme will help you build a good foundation, serving as a great introduction to the strength component of the official Army Fitness Programmes in Part Two (pp.124–147). Each week, there is one workout focusing respectively on the lower body, upper body, and the abs and back (the trunk region), as well as a circuit-style workout for the full body. For every exercise, you can use the "make it easier" or "make it harder" modifications included in the previous pages, to enable you to work at an appropriate level. As with the aerobic start-up programme, there are four workouts each week, performed on non-consecutive days, with a rest day in between. Don't forget to warm up and cool down (pp.96-109) and concentrate on maintaining good technique throughout.

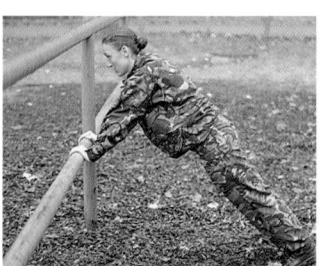

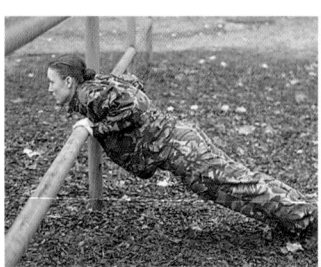

DID YOU KNOW?

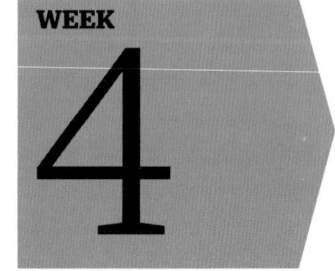

Resistance training doesn't just strengthen muscles, but bones, too. Just like muscle, bones need to be overloaded in order to grow or remain strong, and strength training does just that. Better bone density means a reduced risk of osteoporosis, the bone-thinning disease that affects many women, and some men, in later life.

Session

WEEK

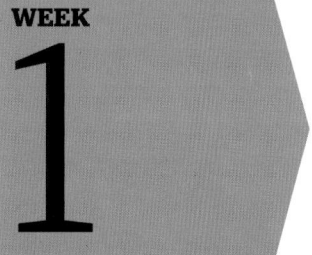
1

WEEK

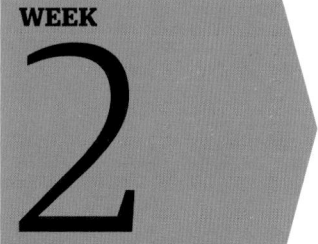
2

WEEK

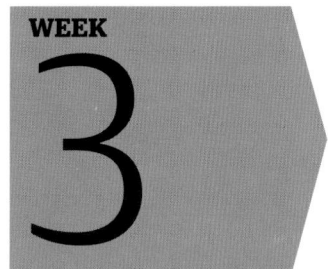
3

WEEK
4

DAY 1	DAY 2	DAY 3	DAY 4
Perform 2 sets x 8 reps of press-up, pull-up, dip.	Perform 2 sets x 8 reps of squat, lunge, step-up.	Perform 2 sets x 8 reps of sit-up, twist sit-up, dorsal raise.	Perform 1 set x 10 reps of each exercise from this week without a break. Rest for 2 mins and repeat circuit.
Perform 2 sets x 10 reps of press-up, pull-up, dip.	Perform 2 sets x 10 reps of squat, lunge, step-up.	Perform 2 sets x 10 reps of sit-up, twist sit-up, dorsal raise.	Perform 1 set x 12 reps of each exercise from this week without a break. Rest for 2 mins and repeat circuit.
Perform 2 sets x 12 reps of press-up, pull-up, dip.	Perform 2 sets x 12 reps of squat, lunge, step-up.	Perform 2 sets x 12 reps of sit-up, twist sit-up, dorsal raise plus 3 x plank (hold for 10 secs).	Perform 1 set x 12 reps of each exercise from this week without a break. Rest for 2 mins and repeat circuit.
Perform 2 sets x 15 reps of press-up, pull-up, dip.	Perform 2 sets x 15 reps of squat, lunge, step-up.	Perform 2 sets x 15 reps of sit-up, twist sit-up, dorsal raise plus 3 x plank (hold for 15 secs).	Perform 1 set x 10 reps of each exercise from this week without a break. Rest for 2 mins and repeat circuit twice.

(REST DAY appears between each of the four day-columns.)

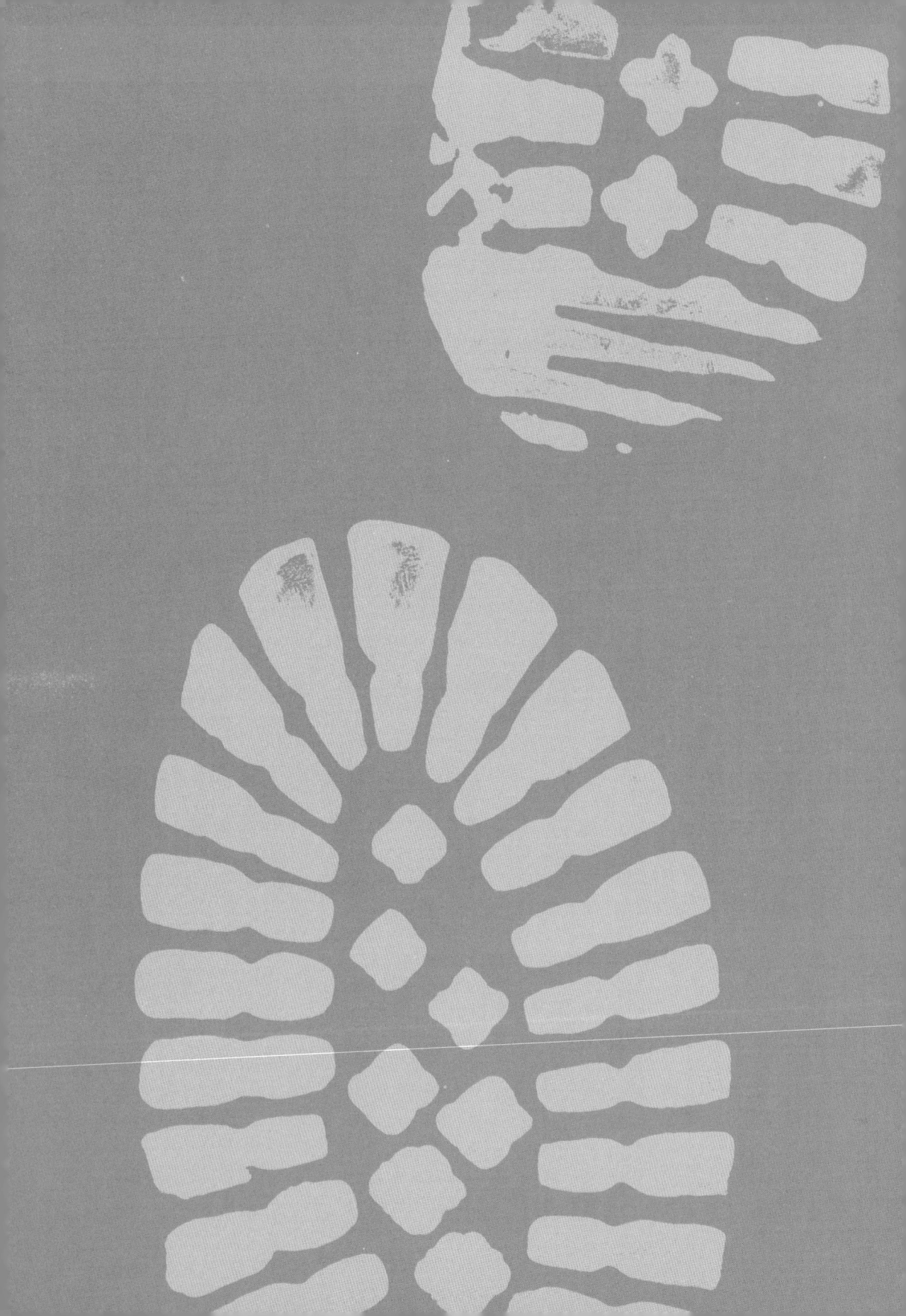

Stretching and flexibility

When muscles are supple and joints mobile, the body is able to move in the way it was designed – quickly and efficiently. A flexible joint can move through a greater range of motion at speed and with ease, leading to enhanced performance, better posture and a reduced risk of injury. That's why the Army now incorporates regular flexibility sessions into military physical training on rest or recovery days, as well as ensuring that physical training is always followed by a cool-down and stretch.

If you are fairly new to flexibility training, the four-week "start-up" programme at the end of this chapter (pp.92–93) will get you going. It will also help prepare you for the flexibility component of the Level One Programme (p.124).

Why stretch?

Physical activity involves muscular contractions in which the muscle fibres shorten. If they aren't stretched out again afterwards, they remain shortened for longer and, over time, can adapt to this shorter length, pulling bones out of alignment (a process known as "adaptive shortening"). Tight, shortened muscles and stiff, creaky joint structures limit range of movement, which can be detrimental both to your general wellbeing and sports performance. Even non-physical activities, such as driving or sitting hunched over a computer all day, can wreak havoc on posture and joint health. Holding the body in a fixed position entails working some muscles more than others, leading to imbalances in their strength and length.

You can see, therefore, why flexibility training is such an important part of any fitness programme.

So what does flexibility training involve?

There are two main forms of stretching: **static** and **dynamic**. As the names suggest, the distinction between the two is whether a stretch is held without moving (as in the splits, for example) or whether you take a joint through its range of motion (such as taking your arm around in a wide circle). **Static stretching** develops what is known as the passive range of motion (your flexibility in a fixed position), while **dynamic stretching** develops the active range of motion (flexibility throughout the full extent of the joint's range). While it is the latter that is important as far as sports performance is concerned, static stretching helps maintain good posture and restores muscles to their resting length after exercise.

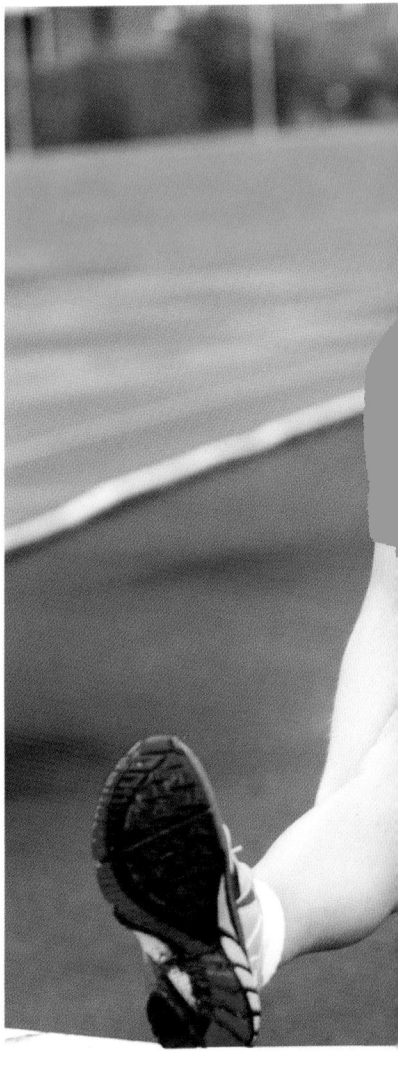

The flexibility regime in this chapter is based on static stretches. Research indicates that the optimal time to perform this kind of stretch is after your workout, when your muscles are warm, pliant and less likely to tear or be overstrained. Stretching straight after the cool-down

PTI Tip

If you perform a flexibility workout as a separate routine, always ensure that you have warmed up thoroughly beforehand, to prevent overstraining or tearing muscles and connective tissues.

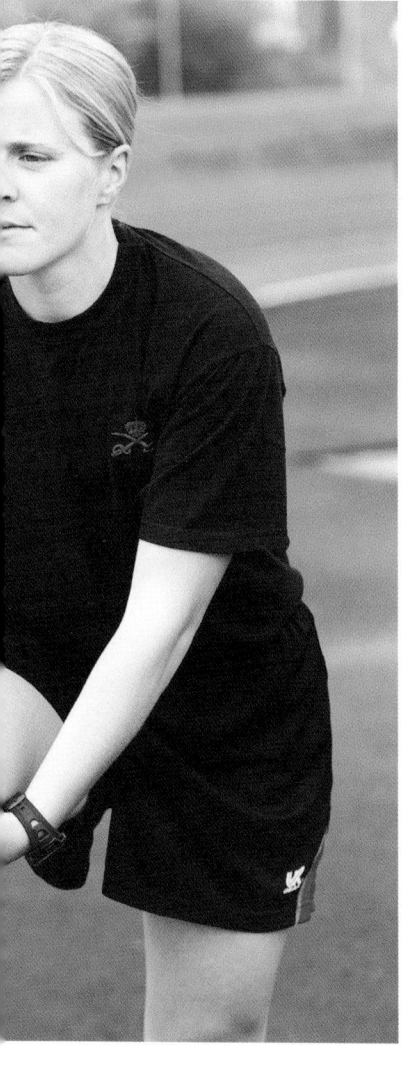

DID YOU KNOW?

When you first place a muscle into a stretched position, muscle "spindles" located among the muscle fibres detect a change in the length of the muscle and report back to the spinal cord. The nervous system then sends a message to the nerves governing these particular muscle fibres to tell the muscle to contract, in order to take it out of the stretched position. This is known as the "stretch reflex" and is the reason why you need to hold a stretch for a few seconds, in order to override this protective mechanism.

flexibility. Try to put aside some time to go through a comprehensive flexibility workout once or twice a week, based on the stretch routine shown over the following pages. But remember, improvements in flexibility come gradually, and will be lost if stretching is not regularly maintained.

Six good reasons to stretch

Stretching:

- Speeds up the removal of waste products and the arrival of fresh nutrients to muscles post-workout.
- Increases blood supply to joint structures, keeping them healthy and mobile.
- Hastens the return of muscles to "resting" length.
- Improves mobility so that day-to-day activities, such as reaching up to a high shelf or taking your arms behind your back, become easier.
- Slows down the decline in flexibility that occurs as we age (a recent study at the University of Nevada concluded that stiffness and lack of flexibility was more a result of lack of use than of age per se).
- Allows you to take some "time out" and can be an aid to relaxation.

section of your workout (see p.108) helps the muscles relax and return to their resting length, "undoing" the muscular shortening caused by physical activity and helping to speed up recovery.

Static stretching can also be valuable as a stand-alone workout. That is because while a brief post-workout stretch will assist in maintaining your current range of movement, it is not sufficient to develop and enhance flexibility. In a "pure flexibility" session, the stretches are held for longer and repeated more frequently, as the goal is to actually develop and increase

Full body stretch

The stretch regime shown here will stretch all the major muscles in the body, helping you to remain supple and mobile.

1. NECK

Stand tall and bend the head directly to the side, to stretch out the side of the neck.

To increase the stretch, take your hand over your head and gently pull the head further to the side.

How to stretch

- Only stretch muscles that are thoroughly warm.
- Stay relaxed and breathe freely.
- Slowly lengthen the muscle towards the limit of your pain-free range. It should be a sensation of slight discomfort, not pain.
- Concentrate on correct body alignment. Know which muscle or muscle group you are stretching.
- Do not jerk or bounce – keep movements slow and controlled.
- For a post-workout stretch, hold the stretch for 10–15 seconds. You should feel it "give" or relax a little. When you do, you can extend a little further into the stretch and hold for a further 10–15 seconds. Repeat each stretch at least twice.
- For a stand-alone flexibility session, hold each stretch for up to 60 seconds and repeat 3–4 times.
- Remember to stretch both sides or limbs.
- Wear loose, comfortable clothing to stretch in. You can stretch with bare feet if you prefer.

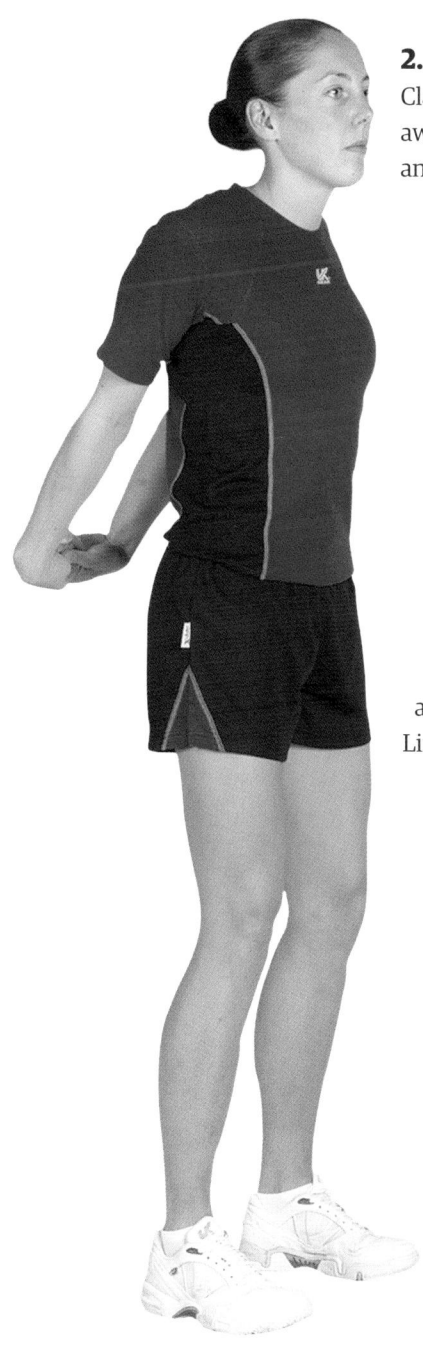

2. CHEST

Clasp your hands behind your back and gently pull the arms away from the back, keeping your arms as straight as possible and the shoulders down.

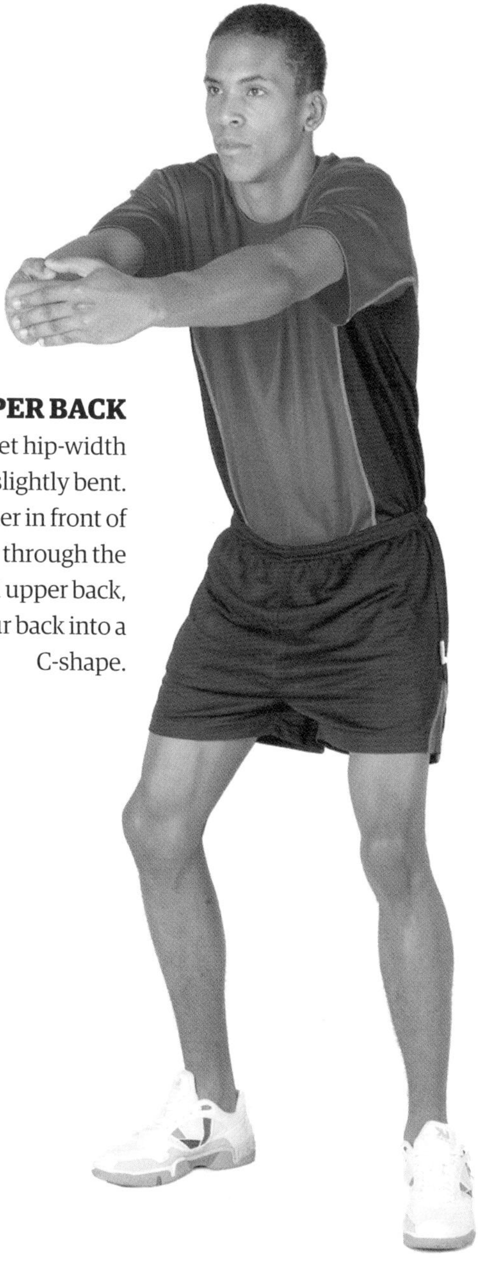

3. UPPER BACK

Stand with feet hip-width apart and knees slightly bent. Link hands together in front of you. Push away through the shoulders and upper back, rounding your back into a C-shape.

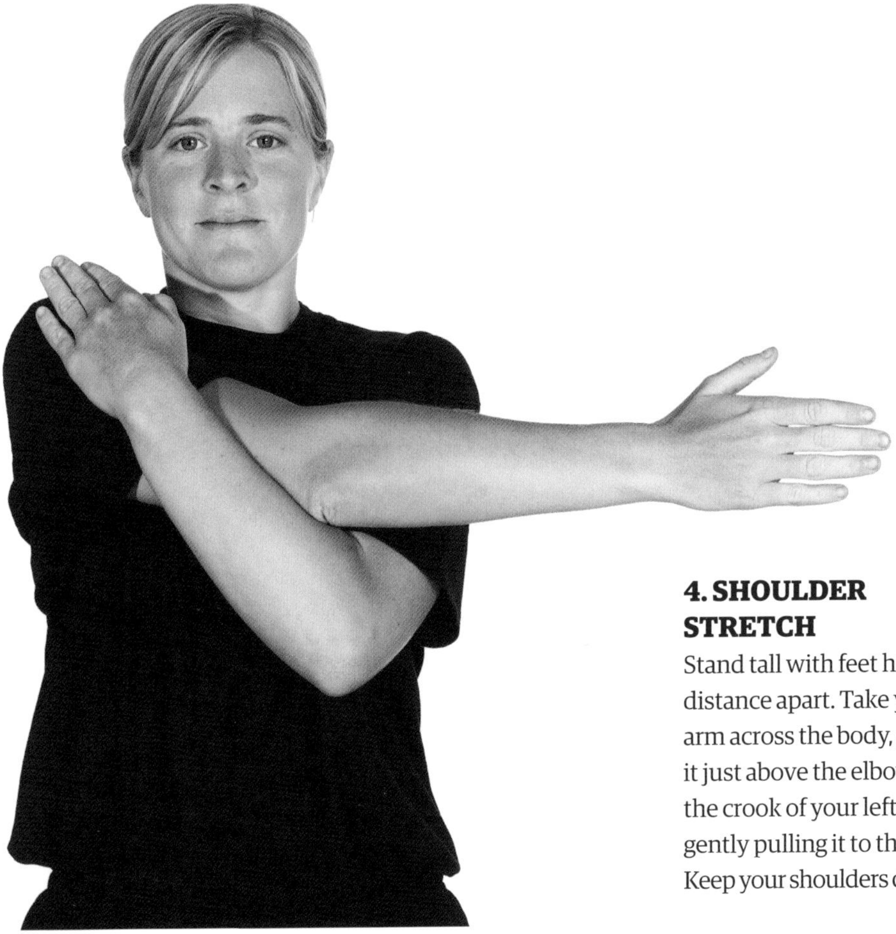

4. SHOULDER STRETCH

Stand tall with feet hip-distance apart. Take your right arm across the body, grasping it just above the elbow with the crook of your left arm and gently pulling it to the chest. Keep your shoulders down.

5. KNEELING SHOULDER STRETCH

To stretch the front and middle of the shoulders, go on to all fours, sit back on your haunches and bend your torso forward, extending your arms out on the floor in front of you.

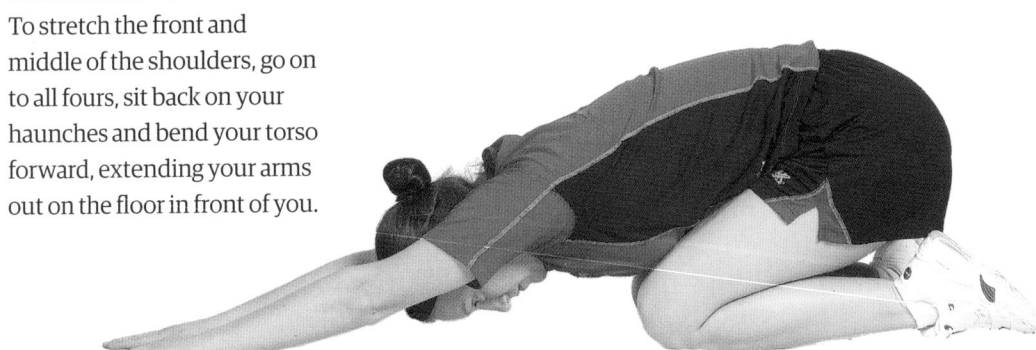

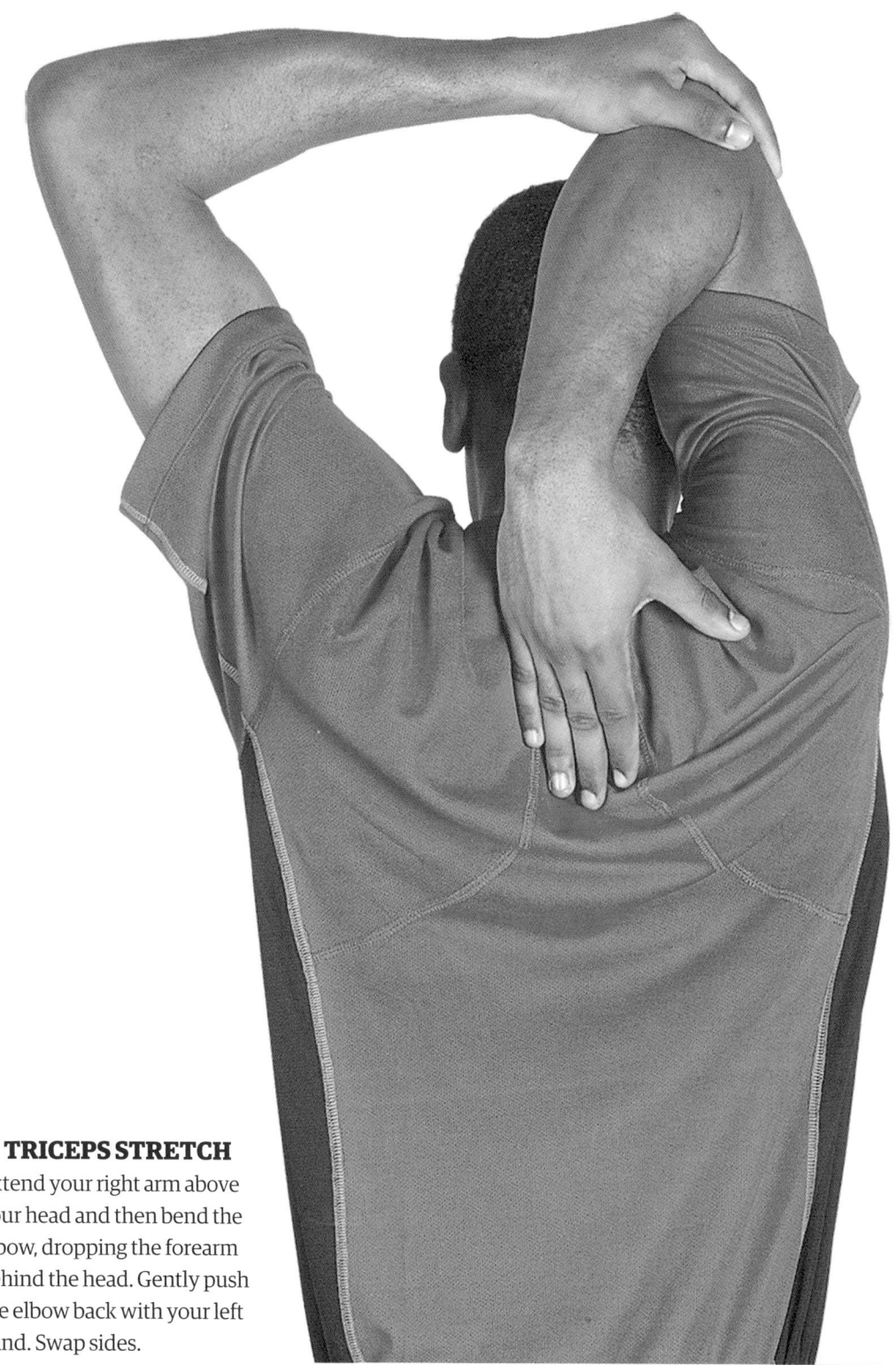

6. TRICEPS STRETCH

Extend your right arm above your head and then bend the elbow, dropping the forearm behind the head. Gently push the elbow back with your left hand. Swap sides.

7. FOREARM AND WRIST STRETCH

Extend both arms out in front - turning the right hand upwards and using the left hand to gently press the fingers away. Feel a stretch along the underside of the arm and wrist. Swap sides.

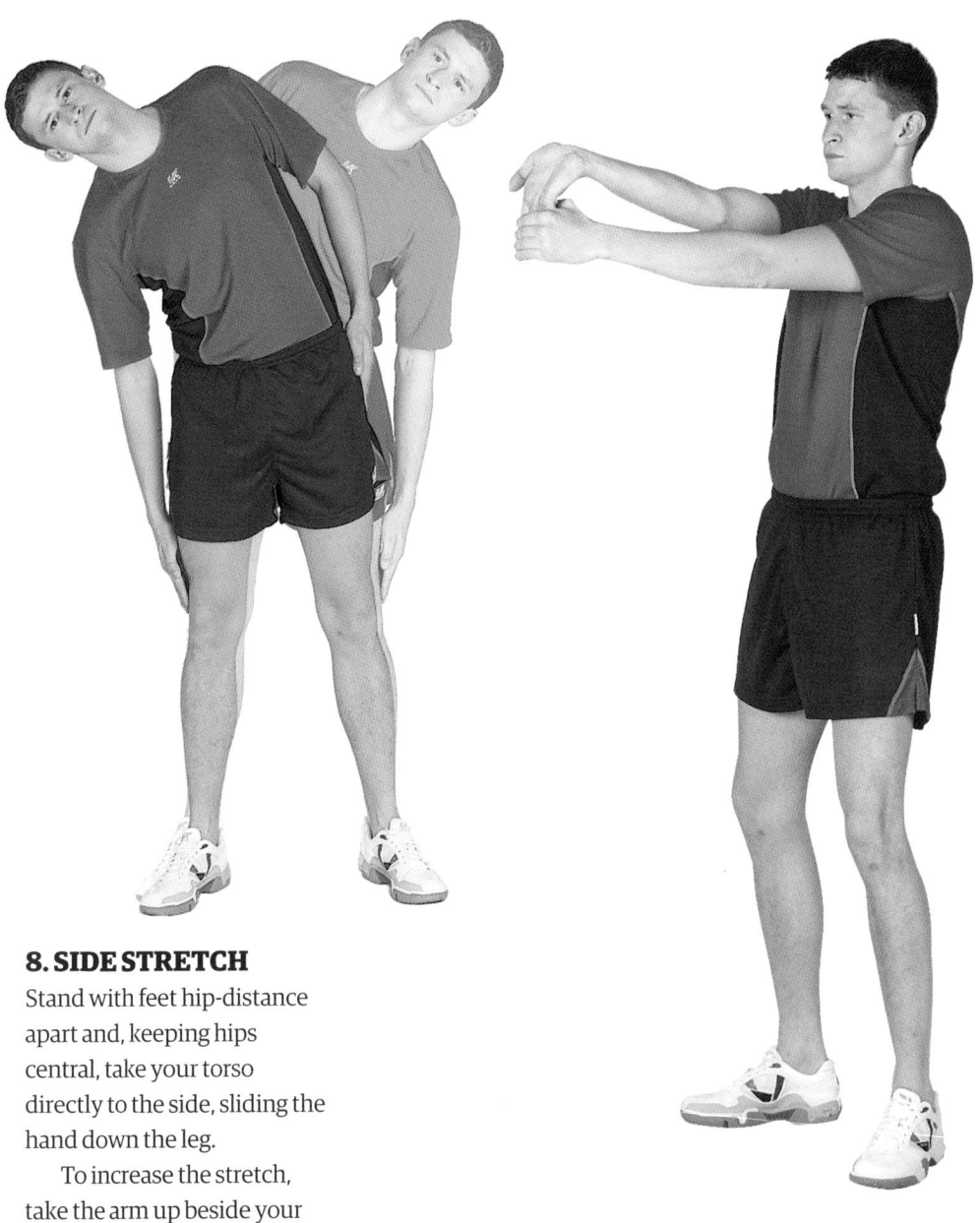

8. SIDE STRETCH

Stand with feet hip-distance apart and, keeping hips central, take your torso directly to the side, sliding the hand down the leg.

To increase the stretch, take the arm up beside your ear. Swap sides.

9. LOWER BACK STRETCH

Lie on the floor and bring your knees into your chest, grasping hold of your shins to increase the stretch.

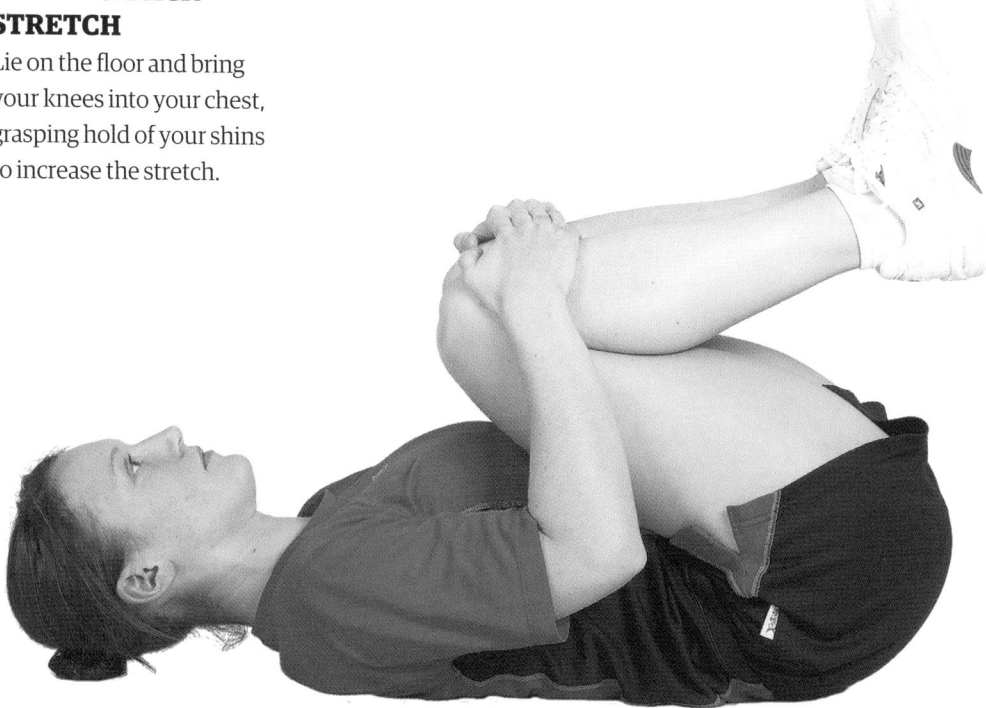

10. MODIFIED COBRA

Lie face down on the floor and raise yourself up on your forearms, elbows below shoulders, forearms pointing forwards. Press your hipbones into the floor and allow your back to extend, looking forwards and not up or down.

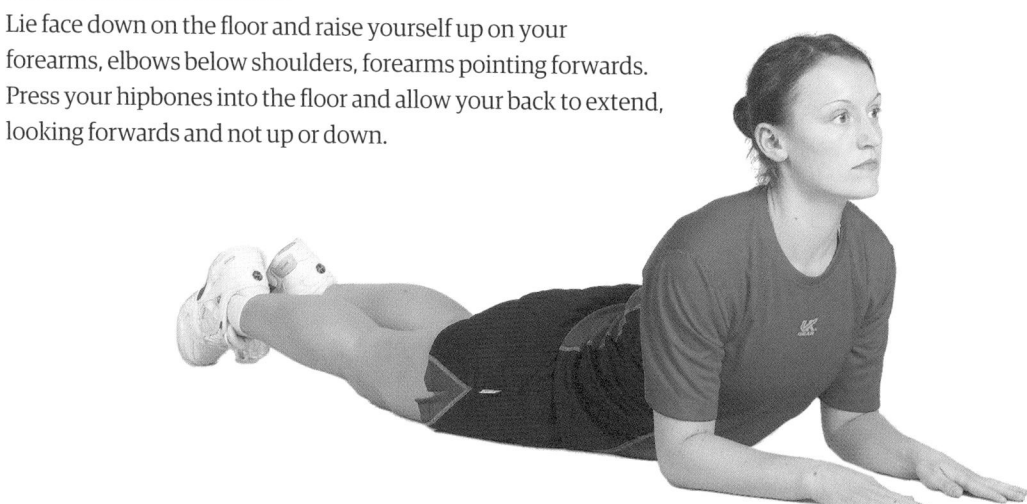

11-12. CALF STRETCHES

Take a big step (about 1 metre) forward with your left leg, keep your right leg straight, pressing the heel down to the floor (right).

Bend the left knee and press the hips forward. Ensure the foot is in line with the leg. Swap sides.

Now bring the back leg closer to the front, and bend both knees, to stretch the lower part of the back calf (below). Swap sides.

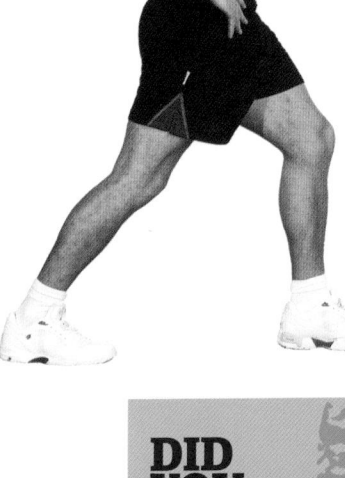

DID YOU KNOW?

Our flexibility declines with age - collagen fibres within the connective tissues thicken and get stiffer, while soft tissue becomes more dehydrated, decreasing joint lubrication and causing "creakiness". Regularly taking joints through their full range of movement and stretches helps slow down this process.

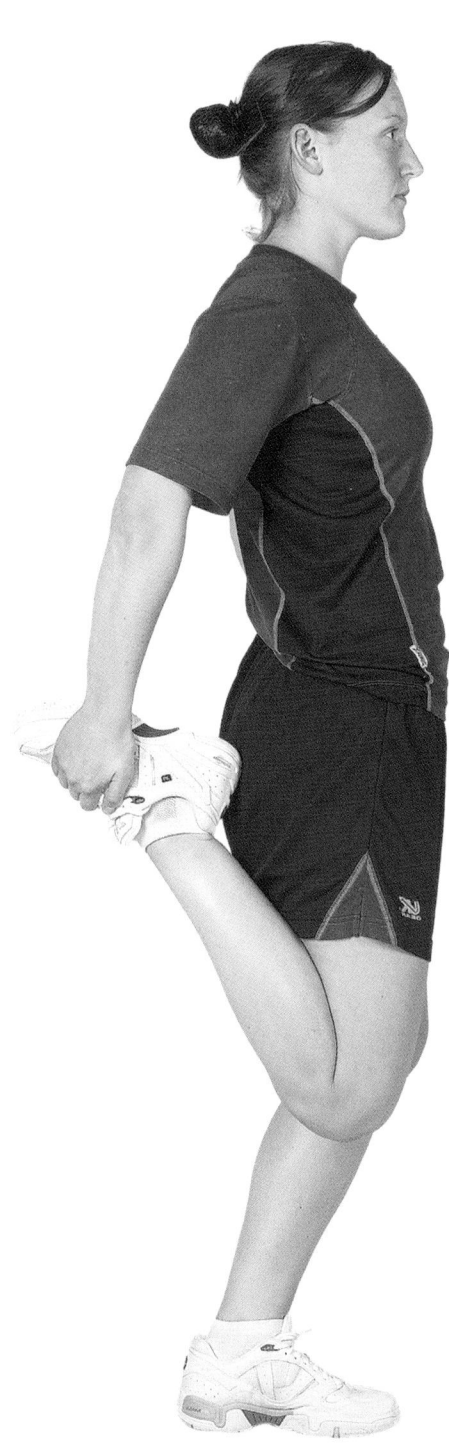

13. QUADRICEPS STRETCH

Standing tall, grab your right foot in the right hand, bending the leg and taking the foot behind you to the bottom.

Keep your legs aligned and don't arch the back or tip the pelvis forwards as you press the foot to the bottom.

14. HAMSTRINGS

Stand tall, and extend one leg out in front of you, foot on the floor, keeping the other knee bent and resting your hands on the bent leg's thigh. Keep the back straight and abdominals gently contracted.

DID YOU KNOW?

At one time, static stretches were recommended as part of a warm-up regime, but more recent research indicates that dynamic stretching better prepares the body for exercise. For that reason, the Army no longer uses static stretches within a warm-up. Although it is not considered harmful, evidence suggests that there is no benefit in performing static stretches pre-exercise, either in terms of injury prevention or improved performance. You can read more about the dynamic stretching or "mobility" exercises used in the Army's warm-up on pages 96-107.

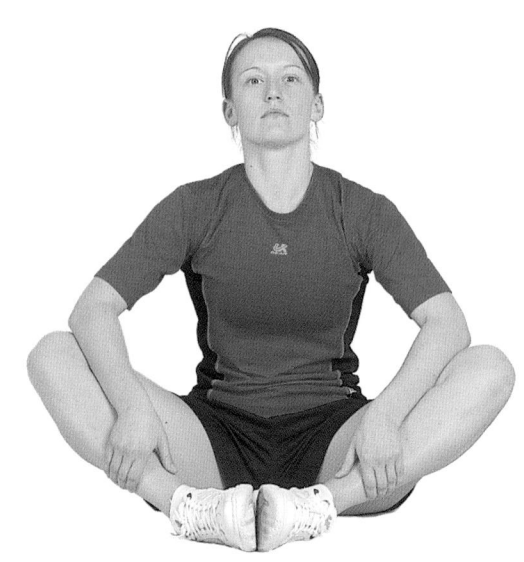

15. GROIN STRETCHES

Sit on the floor and bring the soles of your feet together. Gently press down on the inner thighs with your elbows. Then, extend the legs out straight to the sides, taking them as far apart as is comfortable and keeping the back straight.

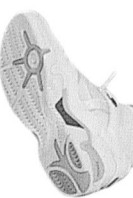

16. HIP FLEXORS

Adopt a lunge position and take the back knee to the floor, shoelaces facing down. Keep the torso upright and lean into the front leg until you feel a stretch along the front of the hip. Make sure the front knee does not extend beyond the ankle, as this puts excessive stress on the joint.

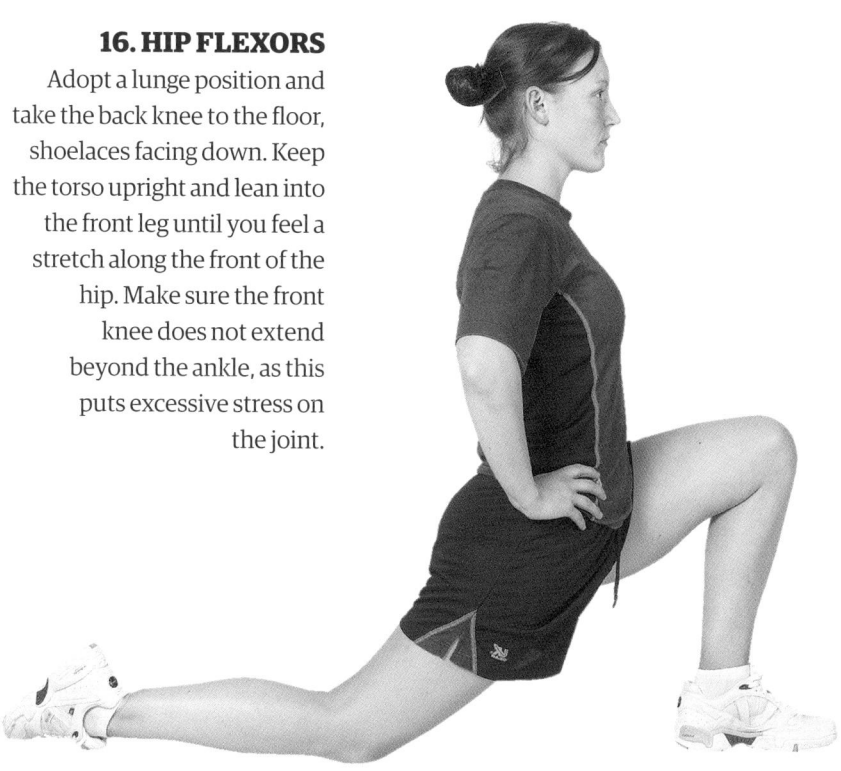

17. GLUTEAL/HIP STRETCH

Lie on your back with knees bent and feet raised. Put your right foot over your left thigh and link your hands behind the left thigh, to gently pull the legs towards your torso and so stretch out the right hip. Swap sides.

Four-week flexibility start-up programme

Haven't touched your toes in years? Struggle to turn around to get hold of your seat belt strap? This four-week programme will help you lay the foundations for better flexibility and mobility, and ease you into the stretching component of the 12-week Army Fitness Programmes (pp.124-147). Refer to the page numbers given for a full description of the warm-ups and stretches to complete.

In week one you will complete the full warm-up (pp.96-107), which includes all parts of the body. This should take around 10 minutes.

In weeks two to four, complete parts 1-2 of the warm-up only, and then perform the specific mobility moves and stretches required for that particular body area (page references are given). The final workout of each week is devoted to a full warm-up and full body stretch. The length of time you hold the stretches for increases gradually as the weeks progress (see the "Session" column).

Session	DAY 1	
WEEK 1	● Warm-up stages 1-3 (pp.97-106)	REST DAY
WEEK 2 Hold the stretches for 15 seconds	● Warm-up stages 1-2 (pp.97-101) **ABS AND BACK** ● Specific mobility moves 9-11 (pp.105-106) ● Stretches 8-10 (pp.86-87)	REST DAY
WEEK 3 Hold the stretches for 20 seconds	● Warm-up stages 1-2 (pp.97-101) **UPPER BODY** ● Specific mobility moves 1-3 (pp.101-102) ● Stretches 1-7 (pp.82-86)	REST DAY
WEEK 4 Hold the stretches for 30 seconds	● Warm-up stages 1-2 (pp.97-101) **LOWER BODY** ● Specific mobility moves 4-8 (pp.103-104) ● Stretches 11-17 (pp.88-91)	REST DAY

DAY 2	DAY 3		DAY 4	
● Warm-up stages 1-3 (pp.97-106)	● Warm-up stages 1-3 (pp.97-106)	REST DAY	● Warm-up stages 1-3 (pp.97-106) ● Full body stretch (pp.82-91)	REST DAY
● Warm-up stages 1-2 (pp.97-101) **ABS AND BACK** ● Specific mobility moves 9-11 (pp.105-106) ● Stretches 8-10 (pp.86-87)	● Warm-up stages 1-2 (pp.97-101) **ABS AND BACK** ● Specific mobility moves 9-11 (pp.105-106) ● Stretches 8-10 (pp.86-87)	REST DAY	● Warm-up stages 1-3 (pp.97-106) ● Full body stretch (pp.82-91)	REST DAY
● Warm-up stages 1-2 (pp.97-101) **LOWER BODY** ● Specific mobility moves 4-8 (pp.103-104) ● Stretches 11-17 (pp.87-91)	● Warm-up stages 1-2 (pp.97-101) **UPPER BODY** ● Specific mobility moves 1-3 (pp.101-102) ● Stretches 1-7 (pp.82-86)	REST DAY	● Warm-up stages 1-3 (pp.97-106) ● Full body stretch (pp.82-91)	REST DAY
● Warm-up stages 1-2 (pp.97-101) **UPPER BODY** ● Specific mobility moves 1-3 (pp.101-102) ● Stretches 1-7 (pp.82-86)	● Warm-up stages 1-2 (pp.97-101) **LOWER BODY** ● Specific mobility moves 4-8 (pp.103-104) ● Stretches 11-17 (pp.88-91)	REST DAY	● Warm-up stages 1-3 (pp.94-104) ● Full body stretch (pp.82-91)	REST DAY

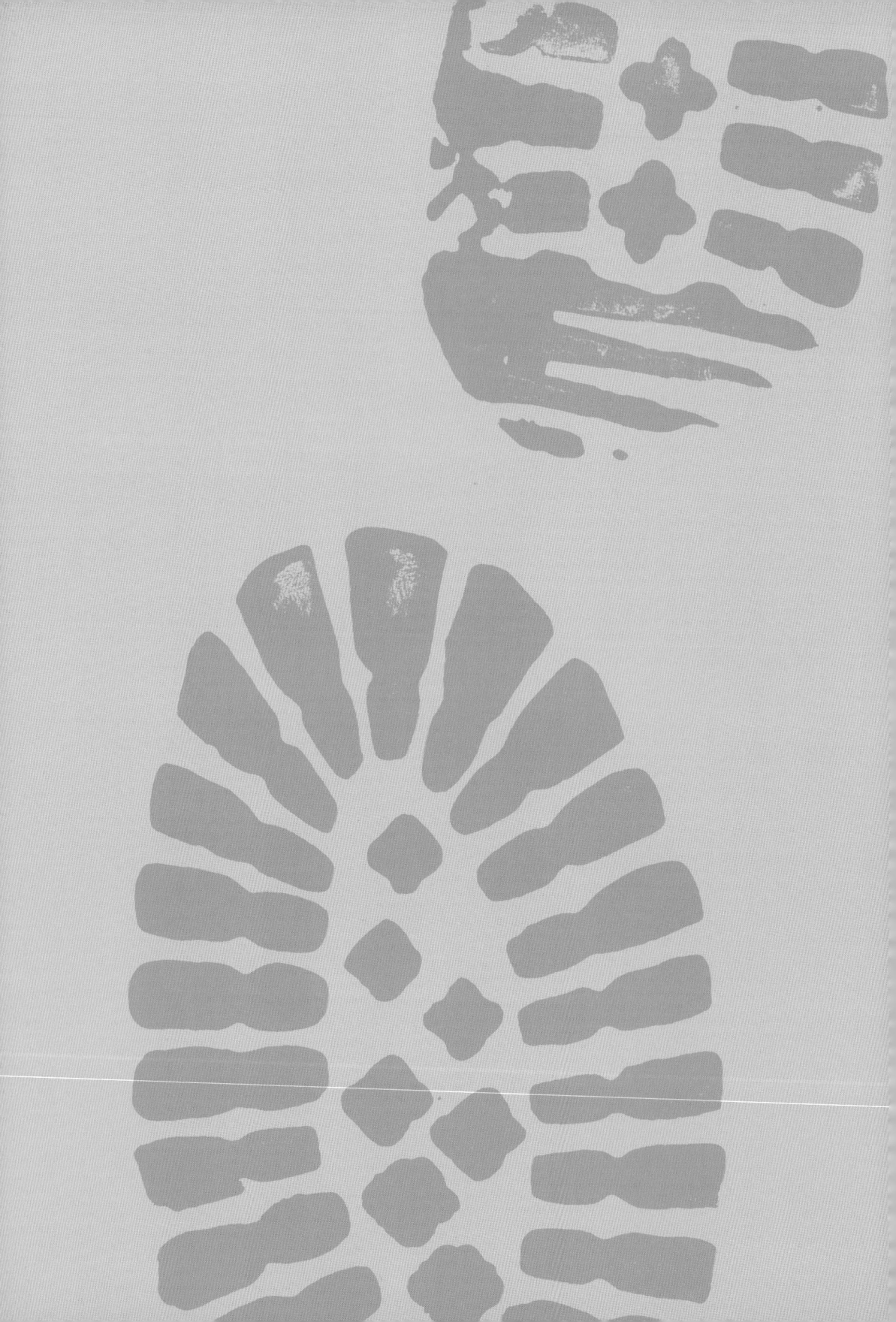

Warming up and cooling down

Warming up and cooling down are essential components of any physical training programme. The purpose of a warm-up is simply to prepare the body, mentally and physically, for the activity to follow. Research has found that a thorough warm-up can help optimise performance and reduce the risk of injury.

At the end of your exercise session, a cool-down helps to gradually return the body to its pre-exercise state – like a warm-up in reverse. Learn how to incorporate these essential practices into your exercise programme over the following pages.

The warm-up

Performed correctly, an effective warm-up can both improve subsequent performance and reduce the risk of injuries such as muscle tears, sprains and strains. It does this by:

- Raising heart and breathing rate, to pump more oxygen around the body.
- Raising muscle temperature.
- Mobilising and lubricating the joints.
- Stretching connective tissue.
- Waking up the neuromuscular (nerve to muscle) pathways, for more efficient movement.

A good warm-up needn't take up too much of your exercise time. In military training, our warm-ups generally take about 10 minutes, but longer, harder exercise sessions may require a little longer. The "dynamic" warm-up used by the Army can be divided into four parts. Static stretching is no longer performed before training, as research suggests that dynamic warm-up methods, such as those shown here, better prepare the body for exercise.

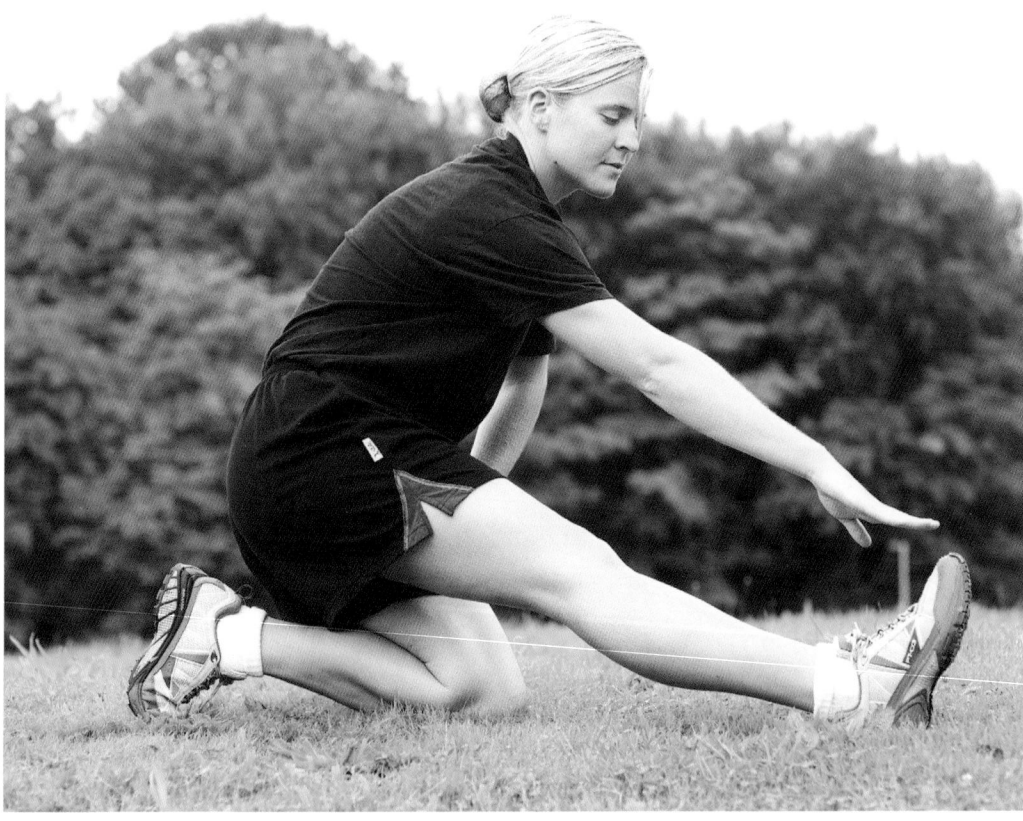

1. Joint mobility

This part of the warm-up is about getting the joints to move more freely by gently bending, extending and rotating them. From a stationary position, work through all the major joints from head to toe. Perform each movement 4–6 times, with each arm or leg where relevant. Continue for approximately two minutes.

NECK

Standing tall, drop your head directly to the left and right sides alternately, and then turn it to the left and right. Gently take the head backwards and drop the chin to the chest and, finally, rotate from the left to right and right to left.

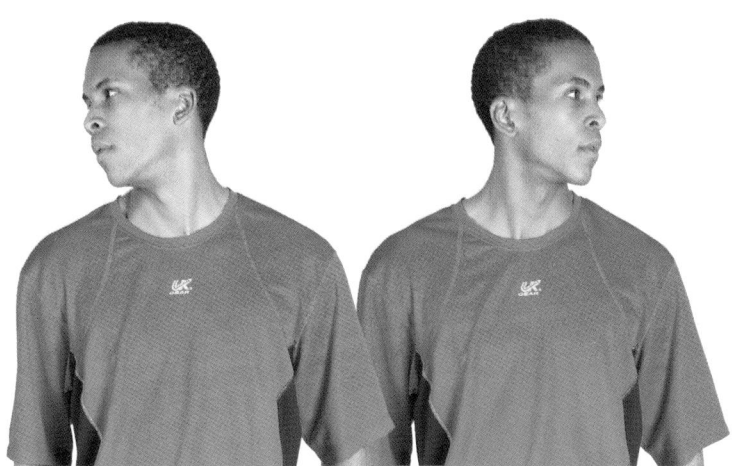

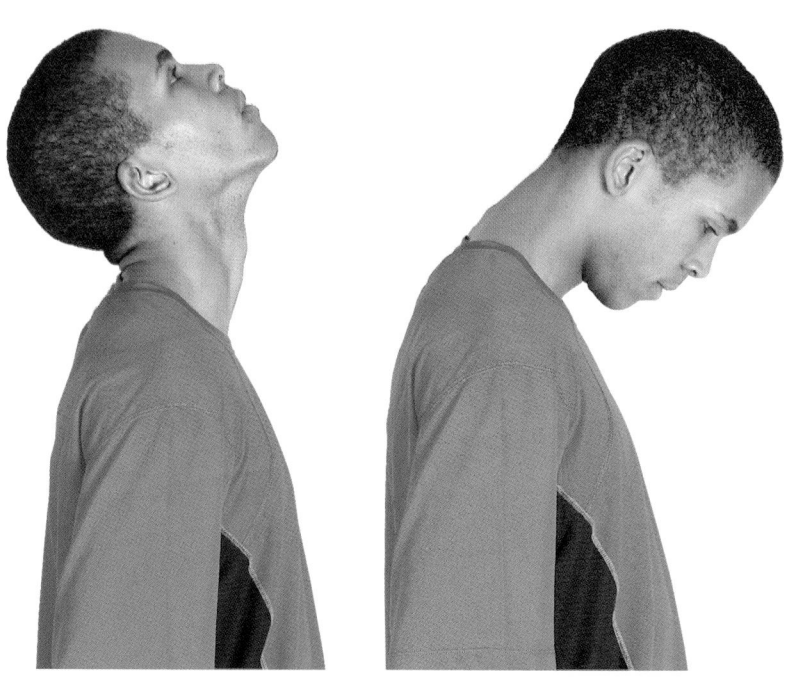

SHOULDERS

Bring the shoulders up to your ears, and then roll them backwards and down. Repeat the movement, bringing the shoulders forward this time.

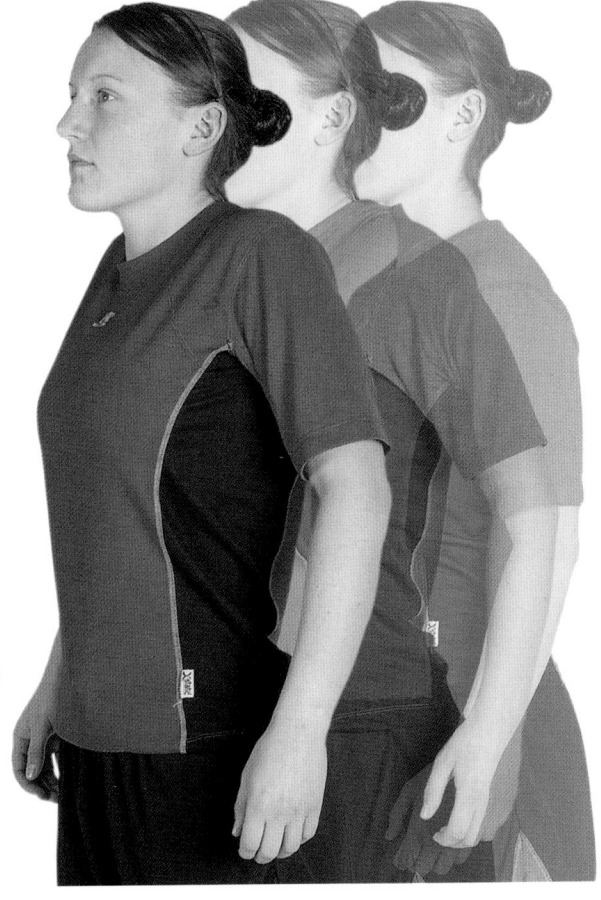

TRUNK

Standing with feet hip-width apart, take your arms to your waist and gently rotate your torso to the left and right, keeping the hips centred. Now drop your hands to your sides and slide the hand down the outside of the thigh, bending the trunk to each side alternately. Again, keep hips centred.

KNEES

Standing tall, alternately bring each knee up to your chest. Next, take your feet up behind you to your bottom. Keep this movement slow and controlled.

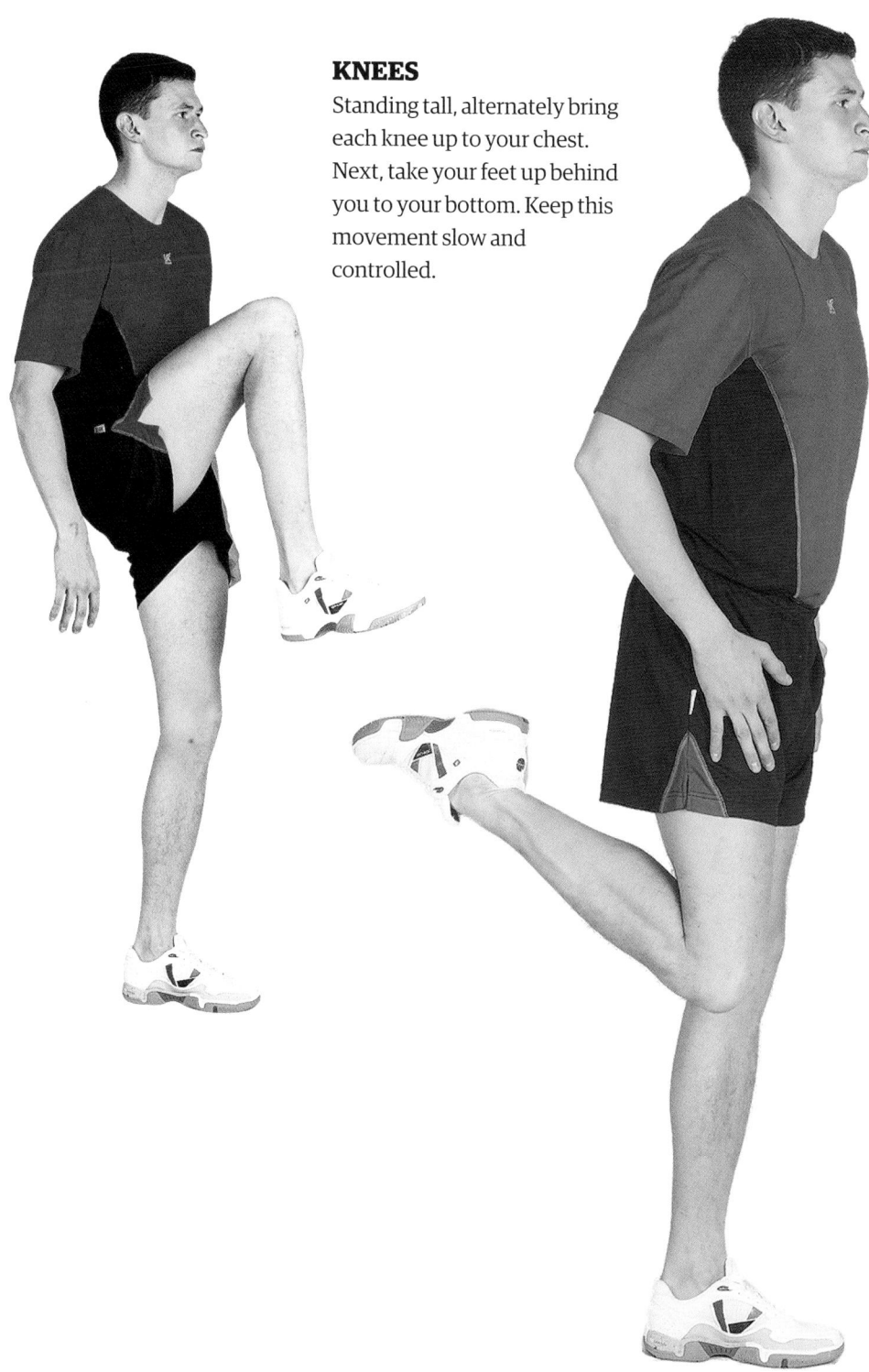

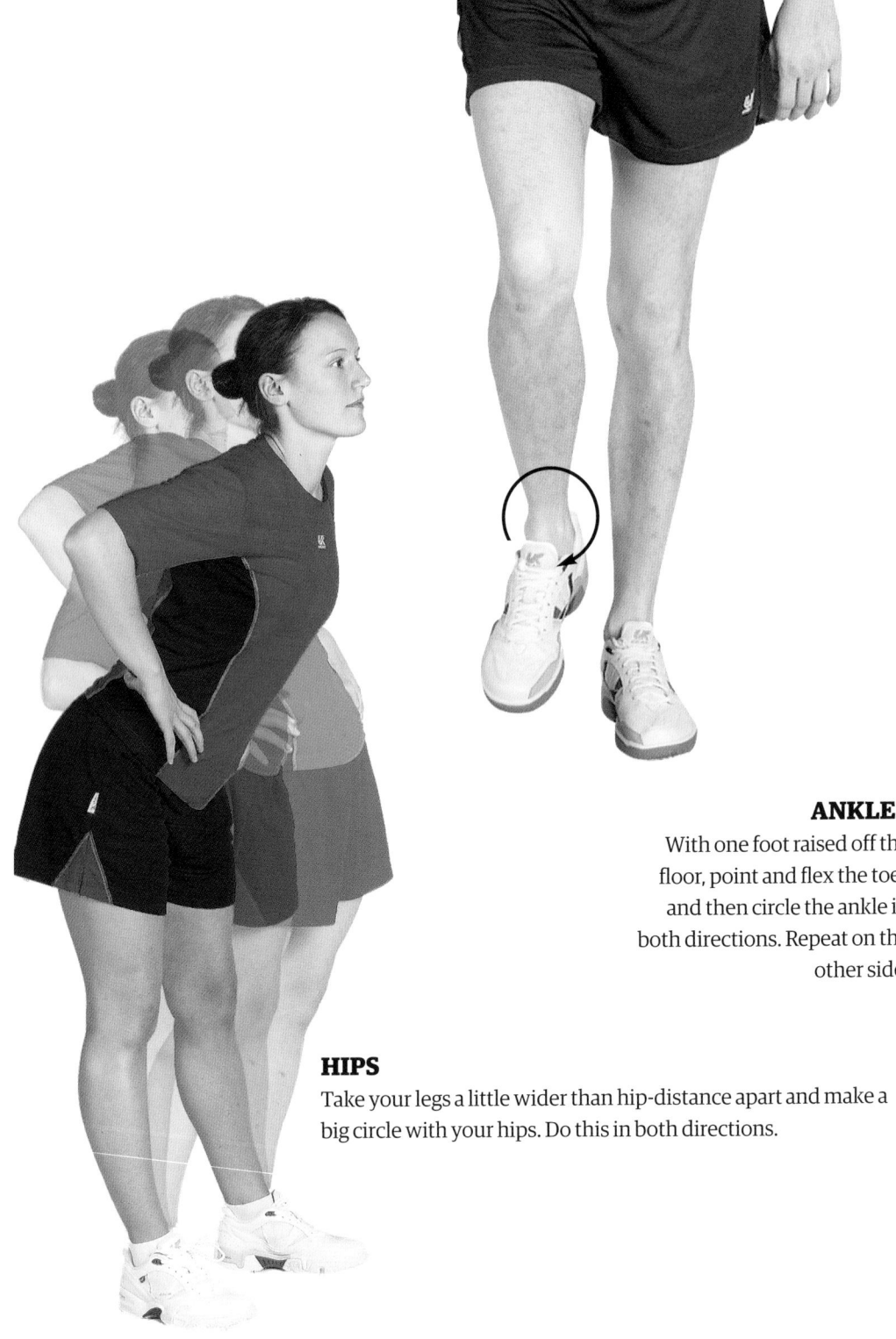

ANKLES

With one foot raised off the floor, point and flex the toes and then circle the ankle in both directions. Repeat on the other side.

HIPS

Take your legs a little wider than hip-distance apart and make a big circle with your hips. Do this in both directions.

2. Progressive pulse-raising

This initial pulse raiser uses large muscle groups in a repetitive movement (walking or gentle jogging is ideal) to get the heart beating faster and to raise body temperature. It can be done inside, for example, simply marching on the spot, or walking forwards, gradually building up to a gentle jog over a 3-4 minute period. Continue for approximately three minutes.

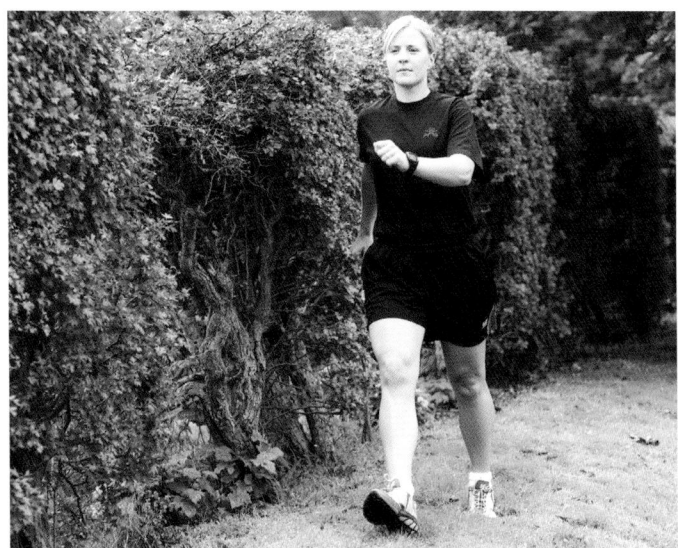

3. Specific mobility

What you do in this part of the warm-up depends on whether you are about to go for a run, take part in a kickboxing class or work out with weights. The exercises involved take the joints through movements similar to the activity you are about to do. For example, to warm the trunk up for a core conditioning workout, you might mobilise the area by doing the hump and slump exercise (p.105). Prior to a run, you might incorporate knee-to-chest and heels-to-bum actions into your warm-up.

The following pages show a selection of specific mobility exercises, indicating which area they focus on. Choose the right ones for the activity you are about to do, performing each one 6-8 times for a total of approximately two minutes.

Upper body

 ARM CIRCLES
Extend your arm straight up to your ear and rotate backwards in a large circle. Repeat with the other arm. Now rotate both arms forwards.

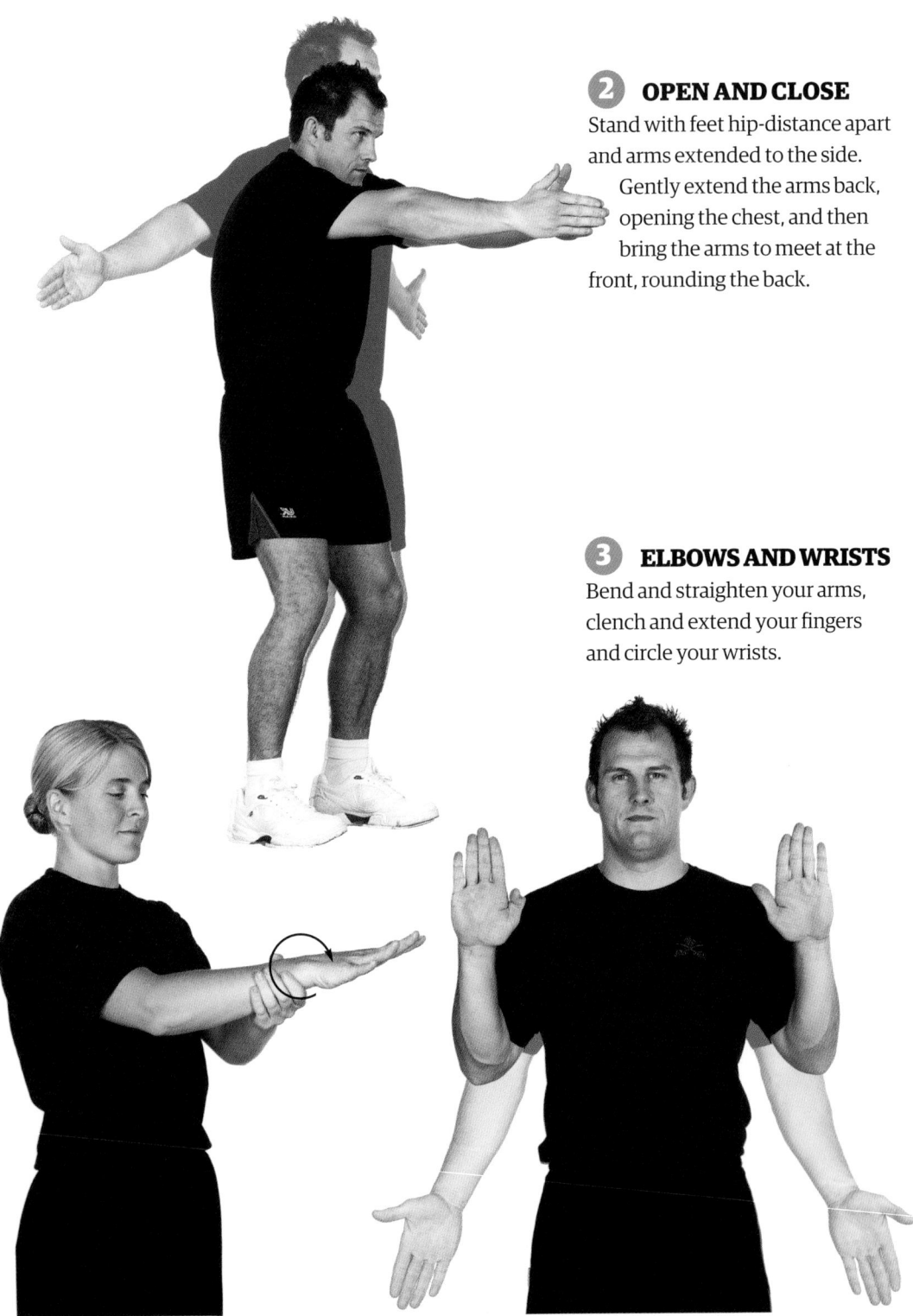

2 OPEN AND CLOSE

Stand with feet hip-distance apart and arms extended to the side. Gently extend the arms back, opening the chest, and then bring the arms to meet at the front, rounding the back.

3 ELBOWS AND WRISTS

Bend and straighten your arms, clench and extend your fingers and circle your wrists.

Lower body

④ CONTROLLED LEG SWINGS

Swing the leg in a controlled manner from the front to the back, keeping the torso stationary. Allow the knee to bend a little as the leg comes to the front.

Now take the leg out to the side and across the body. Swap sides.

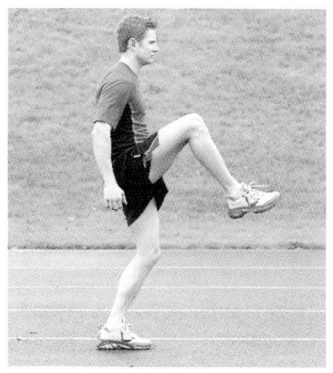 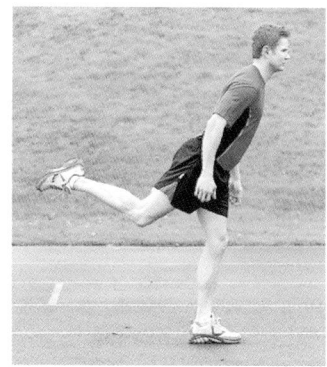

⑤ HEELS TO BUM

Bring alternate heels to your bottom, as in the first part of the warm-up for the knees, but add a jog between each one so that you are bouncing from foot to foot.

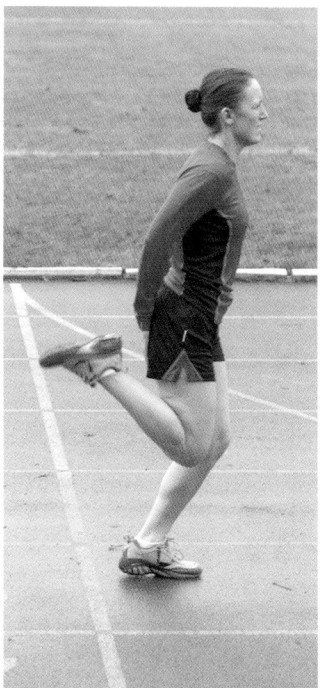

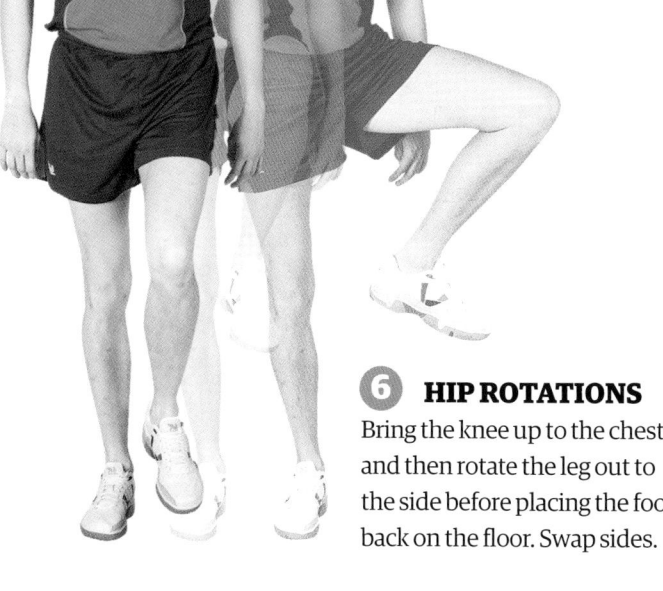

⑥ HIP ROTATIONS

Bring the knee up to the chest and then rotate the leg out to the side before placing the foot back on the floor. Swap sides.

7 KNEES TO FRONT

Bring alternate knees up to the front, springing from foot to foot and keeping the torso upright.

8 WALK ON TOES

Walk forwards, rising up on to the toes from foot to foot.

Abs and back

9 HUMP AND SLUMP
Start on all fours, with knees under hips and hands under shoulders. Start by rounding the back up into a C-shape, letting the head drop down and the neck relax. Then take the spine back through neutral and into an arch, lifting the head and hips. Alternate between rounding and arching.

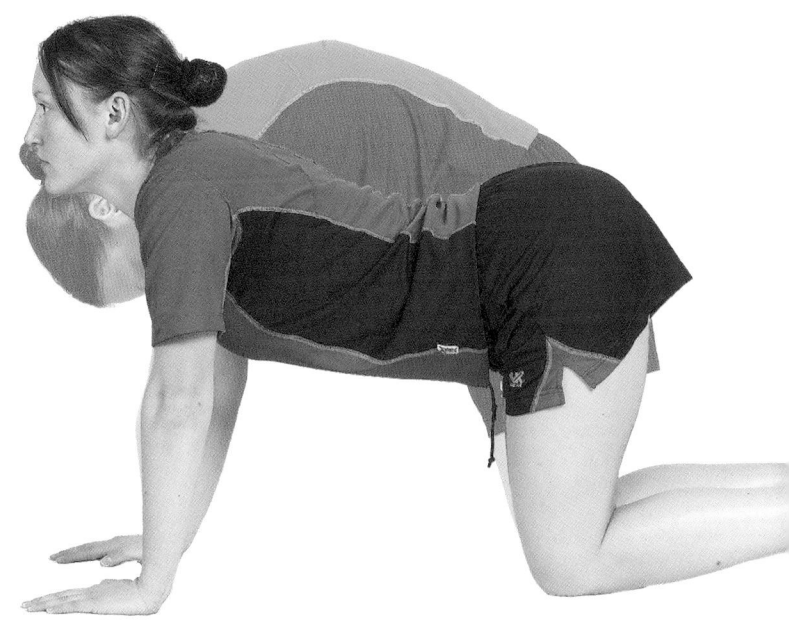

10 TRUNK ROTATION WITH ARMS TO SIDES
Stand with feet hip-distance apart and arms extended to the side and flexed at the elbow. Keeping the hips facing the front, gently twist the torso to the side, leading with the arms and allowing the head to follow the spine. Twist to the opposite side.

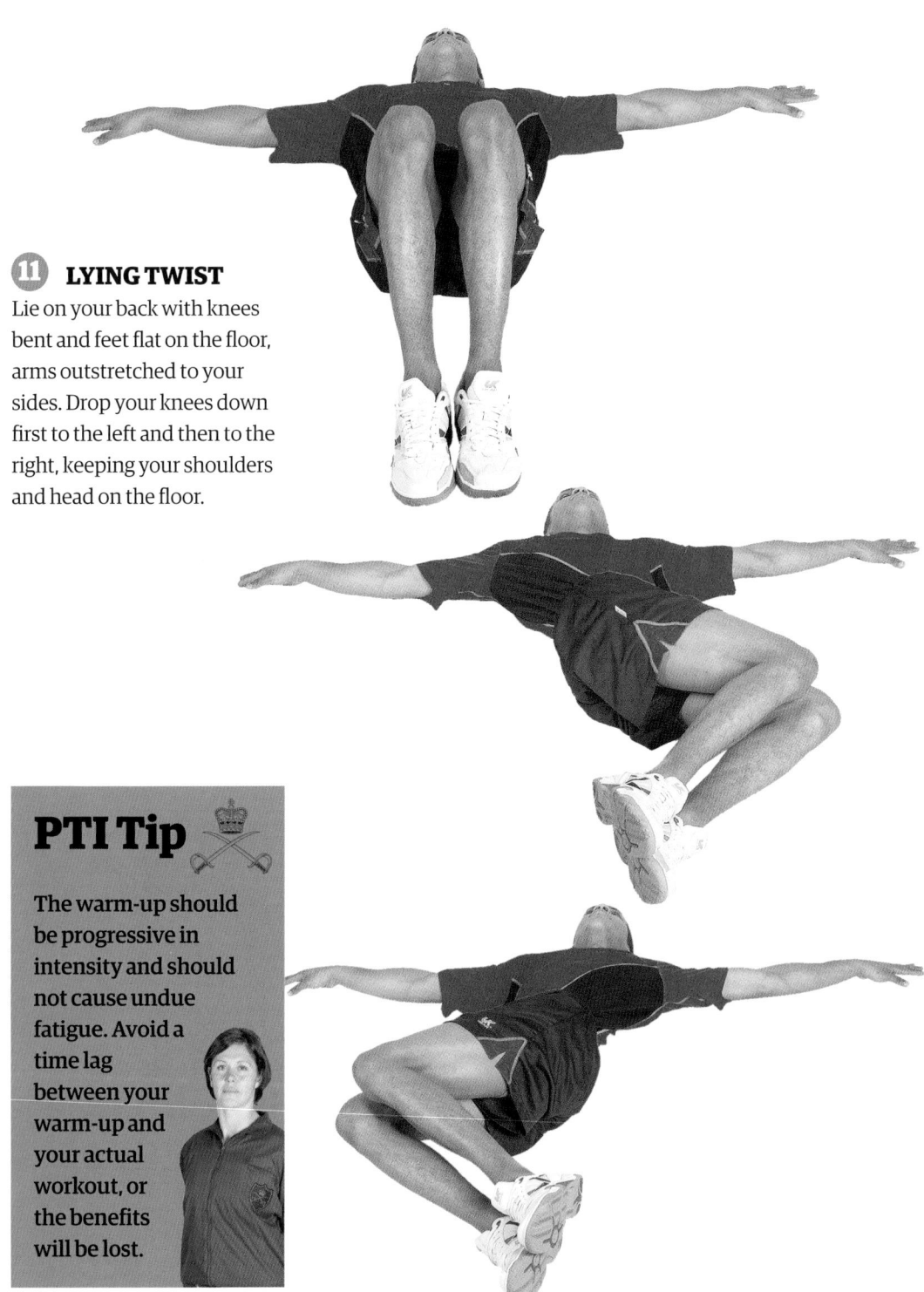

⑪ LYING TWIST

Lie on your back with knees bent and feet flat on the floor, arms outstretched to your sides. Drop your knees down first to the left and then to the right, keeping your shoulders and head on the floor.

PTI Tip

The warm-up should be progressive in intensity and should not cause undue fatigue. Avoid a time lag between your warm-up and your actual workout, or the benefits will be lost.

4. Final pulse raiser

This final part of the warm-up raises heart rate, breathing rate and body temperature further, so you are fully geared up for your activity. Ideally, this pulse raiser should involve the actual activity you are about to perform – for example, if you were going for a long bike ride, you would be cycling, perhaps incorporating some short sprints or hills into the ride. Allow approximately three minutes to get your heart rate and effort up to the level at which you intend to perform the session itself. There should not be any break between the final pulse raiser and the workout.

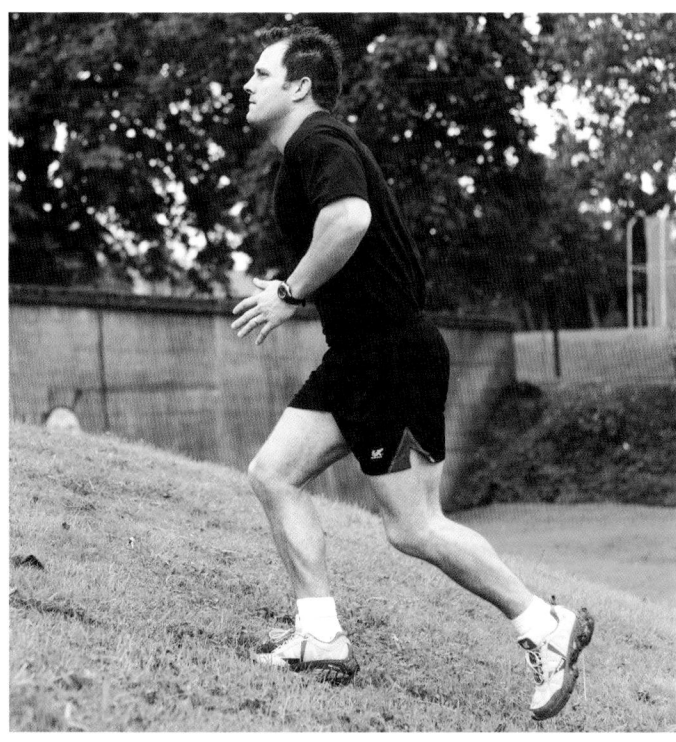

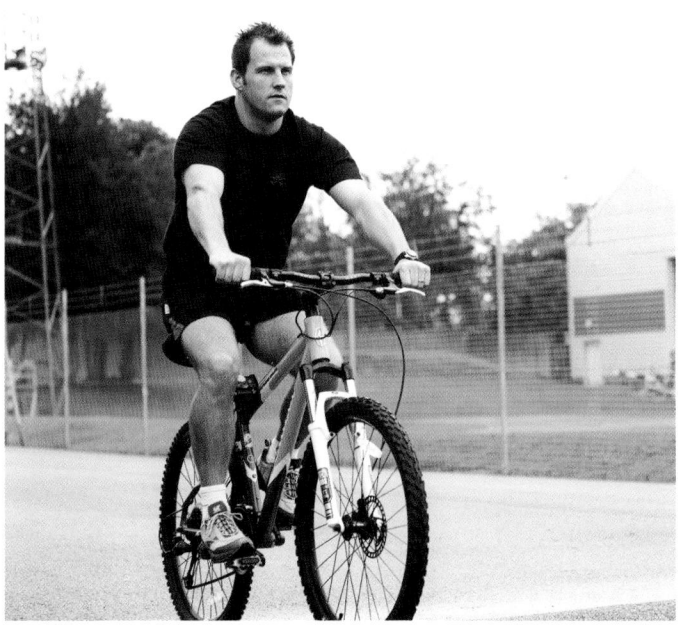

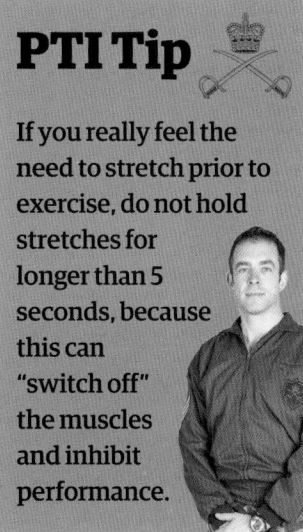

PTI Tip

If you really feel the need to stretch prior to exercise, do not hold stretches for longer than 5 seconds, because this can "switch off" the muscles and inhibit performance.

The cool-down

Cooling down is the most frequently neglected component of workouts. It shouldn't be. If you stop too suddenly once your exercise session is over, the heart continues to pump large amounts of blood to the body, but the absence of activity means that the blood can pool in the limbs, making you feel faint or dizzy. Stopping too suddenly also slows the removal of waste products from the body, hampering the recovery process and increasing the likelihood of cramping and sore muscles.

A cool-down should typically last 10 minutes but can range from 5 minutes to 20 minutes and should incorporate some static stretching to help restore muscles to their resting length. Tailor your stretching routine to the main muscles used throughout the training session, using the regime on pages 82-91 as a reference.

PTI Tip

After a hard session, consume a carbohydrate-based food or beverage within half an hour. This helps maximise replenishment of your muscles' energy stores. Do not wait to refuel until after you've stretched and had a shower.

How to do it

The cool-down should follow on directly from the your workout without a break and, as with the warm-up, it can be divided into stages if you prefer.

An appropriate cool-down will:

- Aid in the dissipation of waste products, including lactic acid.
- Reduce the potential for "DOMS"(Delayed Onset Muscle Soreness).
- Reduce the chances of dizziness or fainting caused by the pooling of blood in the veins.
- Give you a chance to reflect on your session.

1. PULSE RATE REDUCTION

The first goal of your cool-down is to allow heart rate and breathing to begin to return to normal by significantly reducing intensity. For example, breaking into a jog or walk from running (below). Spend 2-3 minutes at this low intensity.

2. JOINT MOBILITY

Next, repeat some of the joint mobility exercises on pages 97-100, focusing on those that target the muscles you've used most in your workout. You can maintain a slow walk or move gently on the spot as you perform these moves. Continue for approximately two minutes.

3. STRETCHING

As body temperature will remain elevated for a limited period, the post-cool-down period is the perfect time to perform your static stretching (see the full body stretch pp.82-91). Hold each stretch for approximately 20-25 seconds and remember to perform the stretch on both sides of the body or limbs where appropriate. Allow at least 5 minutes for stretching.

PART TWO

THE PROGRAMMES

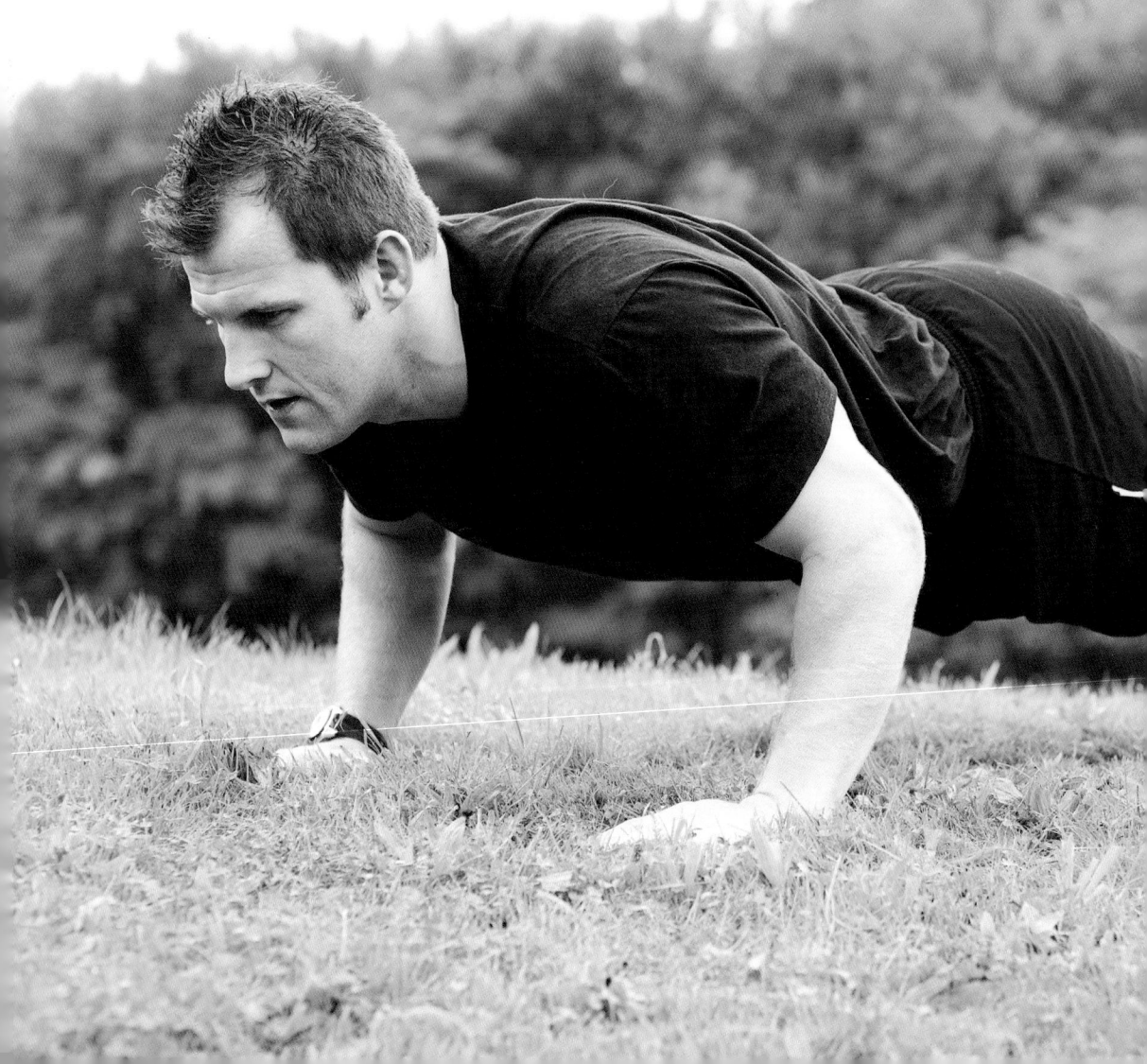

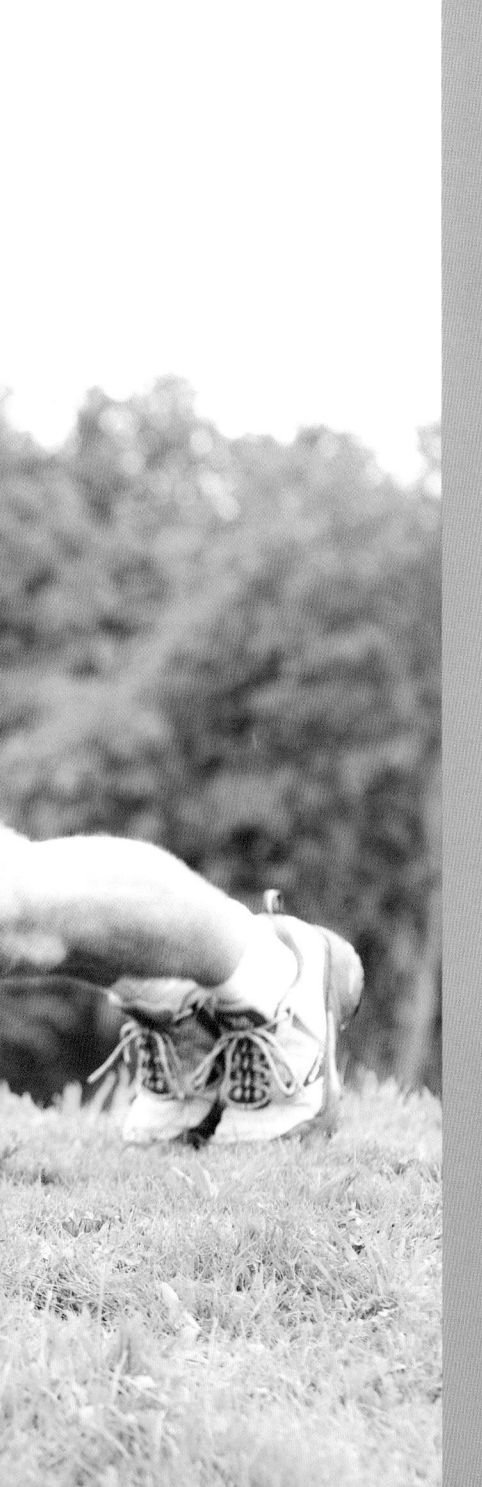

This is where the plan is put into action. The three 12-week exercise programmes in this section are based on those issued to potential Army recruits to enable them to pass basic training. Each of the plans is balanced and progressive, so you can move up to the next one as you complete each level. Make it to the end of the advanced Level Three Programme and you will have achieved a standard of fitness comparable to that of a trained soldier.

In a matter of weeks, you can expect to feel fitter and stronger, with higher energy levels, firmer muscles and less body fat. You will be less fatigued by daily activities, will experience better sleep, digestion and mood and will notice an improvement in your sports performance.

To get a better idea of your current fitness level and ensure you start with the appropriate programme, begin by completing the tests and assessments on the pages that follow.

Assessing your fitness level

The first step of any fitness programme is to determine your starting point, so that you can be sure you are healthy enough to begin exercising and that you work at a level of intensity that is appropriate for your physical condition. Completing the questionnaire and tests in this section will help you assess your current status. And, by repeating the tests at regular intervals, you will be able you to gauge your progress.

Check before you start

Becoming more active is safe for most people, but in some instances it is advisable to check with your doctor before you begin. Start by answering the seven questions below. If you are between the ages of 15 and 69, this questionnaire will tell you if you should consult your GP before you start. If you are over 69 years of age, and are not used to being very active, you should definitely have a health check before exercising.

- Has your GP ever said that you have a heart condition and that you should only undertake physical activity recommended by a doctor?
- Do you feel pain in your chest when you do physical activity?
- In the past month, have you experienced chest pain when you were not undertaking physical activity?
- Do you lose your balance because of dizziness or do you ever lose consciousness?
- Do you have a bone or joint problem that could be made worse by a change in your physical activity?
- Is your doctor currently prescribing drugs (for example, water pills) for your blood pressure or for a heart condition?
- Do you know of any other reason why you should not undertake physical activity?

If you answered YES to one or more questions, talk with your doctor before you start becoming more physically active.

If you answered NO to all questions, you can be reasonably sure that you can start becoming more physically active right now. Be sure to start slowly and progress gradually - this is the safest and easiest way to go.

Delay becoming much more active if:

- You are not feeling well because of a temporary illness, such as a cold or a fever - wait until you feel better.
- You are, or may be, pregnant - talk to your doctor before you start becoming more active.
- You are recovering from an injury.

The assessments

Start your assessment by taking the two measurements given on this page. Then perform a thorough warm-up (pp.96-105) before doing the two-minute press-up test, the two-minute sit-up test, the 2.4-km run and the sit-and-reach test. Take a two-minute break between each test.

Remember to cool down and stretch (pp.108-109) after you have completed the assessment. These tests are scheduled into the 12-week programmes every six weeks to help you monitor your progress. You can record your results for each programme on page 121.

Body Mass Index (BMI)

Calculating BMI is a way of monitoring whether you are a healthy weight. While a useful guideline, it is not an absolute measure of obesity, and should be used with caution. Very fit and muscular people may find that they fall into the "overweight" category because they have a high lean body mass and low body fat (lean tissue being heavier than fat).

To calculate your BMI, divide your weight in kilograms by your height in metres, and then divide this answer by your height again.

Example:
Your weight is 82kg and your height is 1.72m
82 divided by 1.72 = 47.6
47.6 divided by 1.72 = 27.7

BMI classification for men and women

Lower than 18.5	Underweight
18.5-24.9	Healthy weight
25-29.9	Overweight
30-39.9	Obese

Waist-to-hip ratio

Your waist-to-hip ratio is a strong indicator of whether your body weight is healthy. You can work out your waist-to-hip ratio by dividing the measurement of your waist in cm by that of your hips in cm. Measure your waist at its narrowest point – usually around your navel. Next, measure your hips at their widest point – usually around the buttocks. Do not pull the tape too tight when doing either of these measurements.

Men: A ratio of 0.90 or under is desirable

Women: A ratio of 0.85 or under is desirable

Example:
Your waist measures 72cm and your hips measure 94cm

72 divided by 94 = 0.76

Two-minute press-up test

The press-up is a good indicator of upper body muscular endurance, as it utilises most of the major muscle groups in that area. Do as many press-ups as you can in two minutes (find a full explanation of how to perform a press-up correctly on page 42). You may need to take rests during the two-minute period, rather than performing press-ups continuously. Simply record the total number you manage to complete. The chart below shows the number of press-ups you should be aiming for, depending on your age and sex.

Result	Age / Sex							
	Under 30		30-34		35-39		40-44	
	M	F	M	F	M	F	M	F
Excellent	72+	46+	70+	41+	68+	37+	62+	33+
Very good	53-71	30-45	51-69	26-40	50-67	23-36	44-61	22-32
Good	44-52	21-29	41-50	19-25	39-49	16-22	35-43	15-21
Average	34-43	13-20	31-40	11-18	29-38	10-15	26-34	9-14
Below average	0-33	0-12	0-30	0-10	0-28	0-9	0-25	0-8

Result	Age / Sex							
	45-49		50-54		55-59			
	M	F	M	F	M	F		
Excellent	55+	31+	51+	28+	47+	24+		
Very good	38-54	20-30	34-50	17-27	30-46	14-23		
Good	29-37	13-19	a25-33	11-16	21-29	8-13		
Average	21-28	6-12	16-24	5-10	12-20	4-7		
Below average	0-20	0-5	0-15	0-4	0-11	0-3		

Two-minute sit-up test

The sit-up test is a measure of muscular endurance in the trunk region. In the Army's two-minute sit-up test, the exercise is performed with the feet anchored by a partner or low object.

Start by lying on the floor with your knees bent and your feet anchored. Hold your hands across your chest. Maintaining a flat back, curl your head, shoulders and torso off the floor until your torso is in an upright position, then roll back down through the spine to the start position and repeat. Do as many sit-ups as you can in two minutes. As with the press-up test, you may need to take a break between exercises.

Use the chart below to rate your performance depending on your age and sex.

Warning

Stop performing sit-ups if you can no longer keep your back flattened and find it is arching off the floor. Do not perform sit-ups with anchored feet if you suffer from lower back pain.

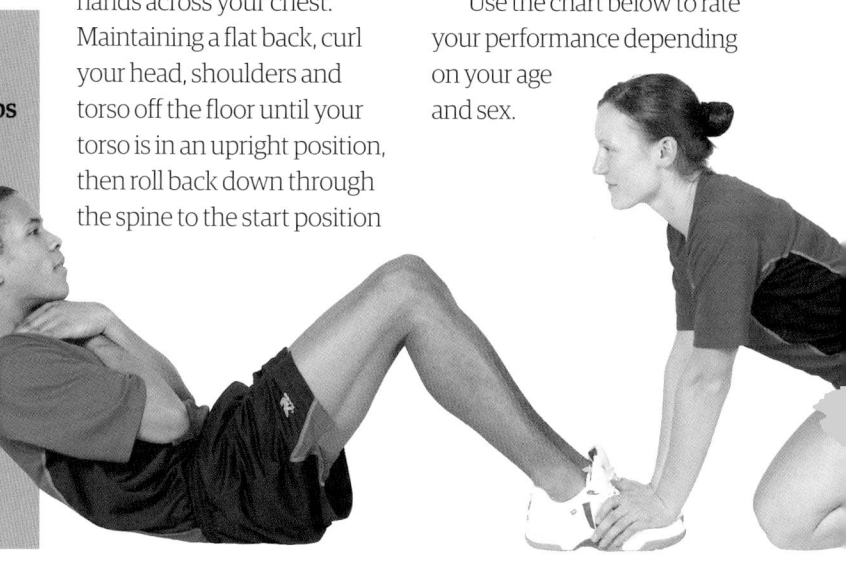

Result	Age / Sex						
	Under 30	30-34	35-39	40-44	45-49	50-54	55-59
	M/F	M/F	M/F	M/F	M/F	M/F	M/F
Excellent	77+	72+	71+	67+	62+	61+	58+
Very good	60-76	55-71	52-70	47-66	43-61	42-60	39-57
Good	50-59	46-54	43-51	37-46	34-42	32-41	27-38
Average	40-49	38-45	32-42	27-36	25-33	23-31	21-26
Below average	0-39	0-37	0-31	0-26	0-24	0-22	0-20

2.4-km (1.5-mile) run test

The 2.4-km (1.5-mile) run is one of the tests the Army uses to assess the aerobic fitness level of all potential recruits. It gives a good indication of cardiovascular fitness and is a good way of monitoring progress, as your pace will increase as you get fitter.

Walk or jog for 800 metres (two laps of an athletics track) to warm up. Then time yourself running 2.4-km (1.5 miles). If you cannot run the whole way, walk where necessary. You can use an athletics track (1.5 miles is 6 laps) or use the odometer in your car to measure the route. Don't worry if the length of your route is not exact – as long as you use the same route next time you can make comparisons.

To see how you fare relative to others of your age and gender, use the table below to benchmark your current performance, set targets and monitor your progress as you work through the exercise programmes.

DID YOU KNOW?

Both men and women need to achieve a 1.5-mile run time of under 14 minutes – less for those who are joining the infantry – before they start basic training. Approximately 1% of the military attain the "excellent" standard, shown below.

Result	Age / Sex							
	Under 30		30-34		35-39		40-44	
	M	F	M	F	M	F	M	F
Excellent	08:15	10:00	08:30	10:30	09:00	11:00	09:15	11:30
Very good	08:16–09:45	10:01–12:00	08:31–10:10	10:31–12:30	09:01–10:40	11:01–13:00	09:16–11:05	11:31–13:30
Good	09:46–10:30	12:01–13:00	10:11–11:00	12:31–13:30	10:41–11:30	13:01–14:00	11:06–12:00	13:31–14:30
Average	10:31–11:15	13:01–14:00	11:01–11:50	13:31–14:30	11:31–12:20	14:01–15:00	12:01–12:55	14:31–15:30
Below average	11:16	14:01	11:51	14:31	12:21	15:01	12:56	15:31

Sit-and-reach test

This version of the sit-and-reach test assesses flexibility in the hamstrings and lower back. Sit on the floor with your legs outstretched, feet flexed and against a wall or other solid object, 20-30cm (8-12in) apart. Reach forwards, fingertips sliding along the floor, and mark the furthest point that you can maintain for three seconds. Roll a pencil along the floor with your fingertips to mark the spot. Ensure your legs remain straight and flat on the floor and do not bounce or jerk to get a better reading. Measure the distance from the wall to your marker to find your result. As your flexibility improves you will be able to reach further.

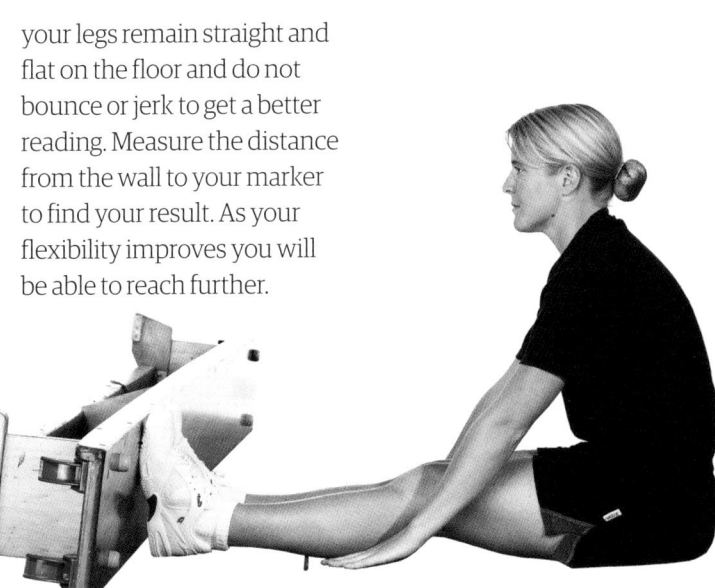

Age / Sex					
45-49		50-54		55-60	
M	F	M	F	M	F
09:30	12:00	09:45	12:45	10:00	13:00
09:31–11:30	12:01–14:00	09:46–12:20	12:46–14:55	10:01–13:10	13:01–15:40
11:31–12:30	14:01–15:00	12:21–13:30	14:56–16:00	13:11–14:30	15:41–17:00
12:31–13:30	15:01–16:00	13:31–14:40	16:01–17:05	14:31–15:20	17:01–18:10
13:31	16:01	14:41	17:06	15:21	18:11

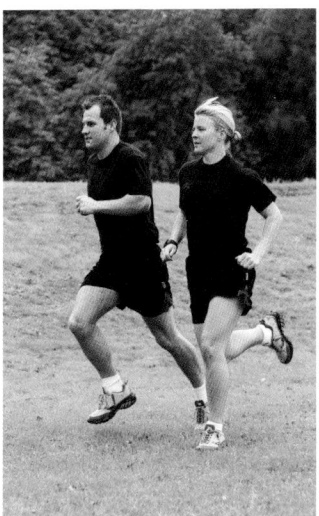

Which programme is right for you?

In order to decide which of the 12-week official Army Fitness Programmes is most suitable, you will need to take into account your existing fitness level and training experience as well as your personal goals and preferences.

How to use the programmes

If you are not physically active, start with the Level One Programme (p.124). If you already exercise 2–3 times a week, try Level Two (p.132). If you've been exercising regularly for some time, begin with Level Three (p.140). Whichever programme you opt for, do not feel that once you've started there's no going back. No exercise programme is set in stone, and you need to monitor how your body is responding and adapt your

training where necessary. There are a few ways to do this. If the programme feels too easy, skip ahead a week. If it is still too easy, skip two weeks, and consider moving on to the next programme. If it feels too hard, repeat the week you found challenging or think about stepping back to an easier programme. All the programmes contain the following five types of training.

Strength training

Perform the number of reps and sets stated, resting for 1–2 minutes between sets. If you cannot make the required number, modify the exercise by using the easier version or do fewer reps in each set.

If an exercise feels too easy, either use a tougher version, select a different exercise for the same body area, or use weights or elastic resistance.

Strength circuits

Strength circuits involve performing a number of strength training exercises in quick succession. This introduces an element of aerobic training into the session. Perform the exercises with a 20-second rest between each and, where relevant, a 2-minute rest between each circuit. If that feels too easy, reduce the amount of rest to 10 seconds between each exercise and 1 minute between circuits.

Aerobic training

When performing the aerobic training sessions, use the table on page 27 to remind yourself of how the effort level stipulated should feel.

Flexibility training

When flexibility training is part of a training session, remember to hold each

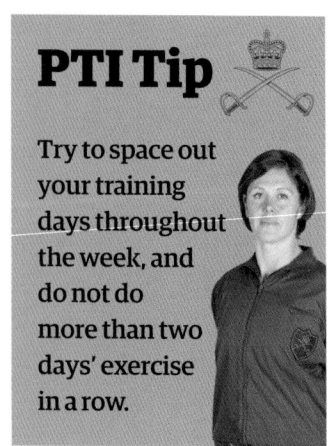

PTI Tip

Try to space out your training days throughout the week, and do not do more than two days' exercise in a row.

PTI Tip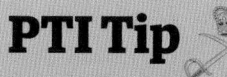

If you're short of time and are tempted to skip your post-workout stretch, concentrate just on the muscle groups specific to the activity you have just performed. For example, the lower body muscles if you've been for a run, or the upper body if you've performed upper body strength training.

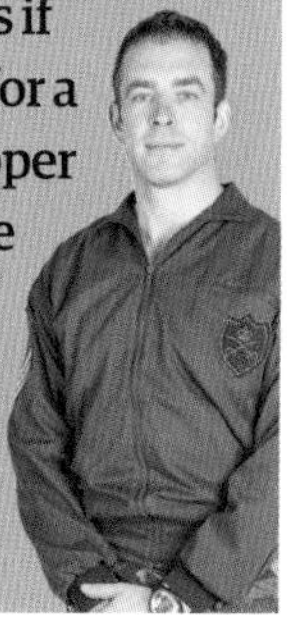

stretch for 10-15 seconds (on each limb or side, where relevant) and perform each stretch twice. Do not bounce in and out of the stretch - hold a static position.

Sport/cross training

Some sessions within the 12-week programmes are dedicated to a sport of your choice such as swimming or cycling. This cross training (see p.154) adds some variety to your regime and gives you the opportunity to try new activities, or rediscover old ones.

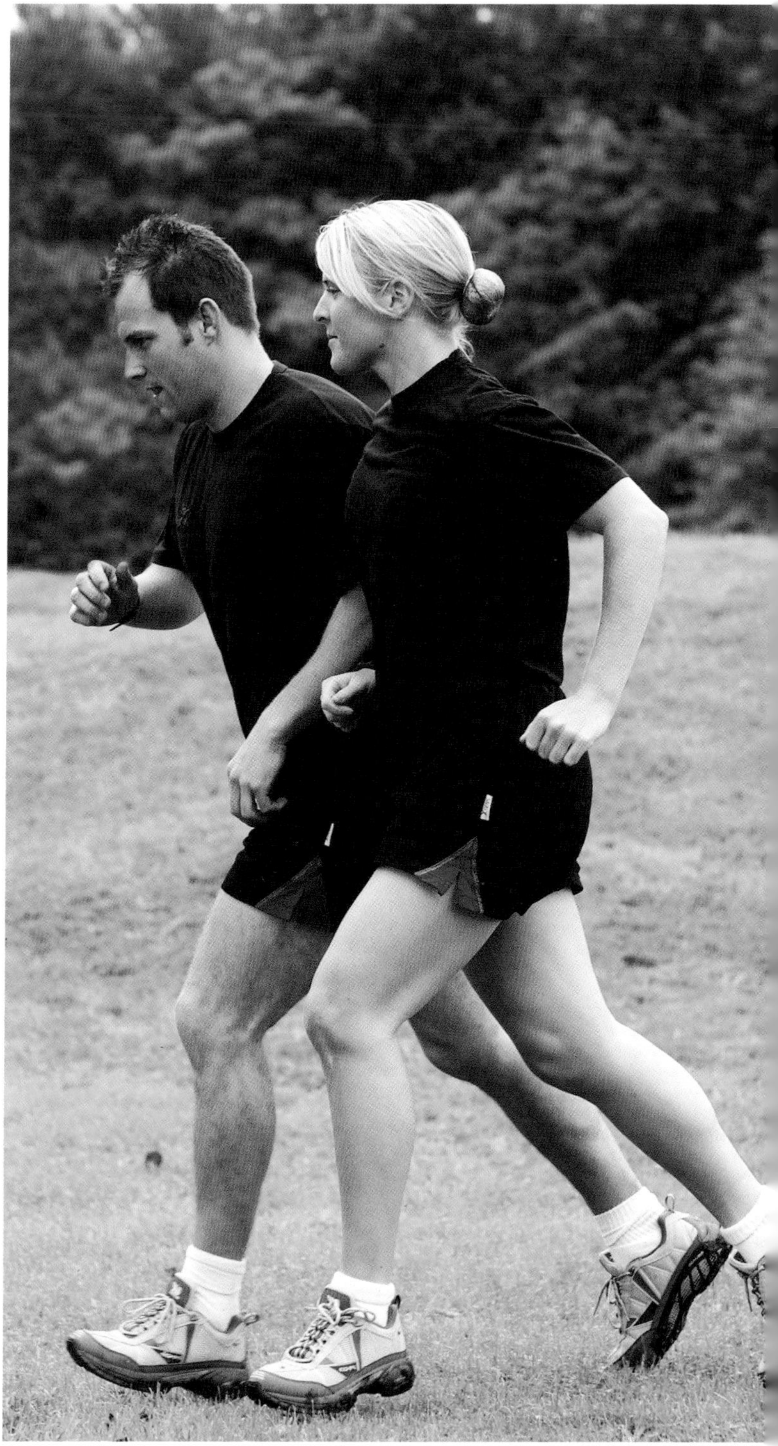

Your personal results log

Use the tables opposite to keep a written record of your progress as you work through the different programme levels.

Before you begin a programme, perform the group of tests described on pages 113 to 117 and write down your results in the first row (Week 1) of the tables. The tests are repeated six weeks into each programme and again at the end of each 12-week block, so by recording your results here you will build up a good picture of your progress. Don't forget to start every exercise session with a warm-up and finish with a cool-down and stretch as shown on pages 97-109.

PTI Tip

Remember to use good technique when you are performing the exercises - and do not continue if you cannot do so without losing form. Quality is more important than quantity.

DID YOU KNOW?

It takes approximately six weeks to see results from fitness training. But you'll probably be feeling the benefits more quickly.

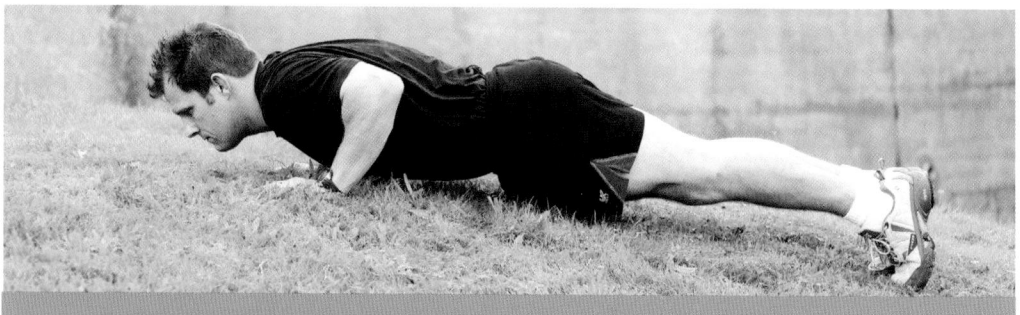

Key terms used in the programmes

reps - the number of repetitions of that particular activity or exercise to perform

% effort - a measure of the level at which you feel you are working (see p.27)

recovery - the period in between efforts or reps when you can get your breath back

rest day - a day on which you do not perform any physical activity, to allow your body to recover. You can perform stretches on these days.

steady state run - jogging or running at an even, comfortable pace.

Level One

	Date	BMI	Waist-to-hip ratio	2-minute press-up test	2-minute sit-up test	1.5-mile run test	sit-and-reach test
week 1							
week 6							
week 12							

Level Two

	Date	BMI	Waist-to-hip ratio	2-minute press-up test	2-minute sit-up test	1.5-mile run test	sit-and-reach test
week 1							
week 6							
week 12							

Level Three

	Date	BMI	Waist-to-hip ratio	2-minute press-up test	2-minute sit-up test	1.5-mile run test	sit-and-reach test
week 1							
week 6							
week 12							

Quick Exercise Reference Guide

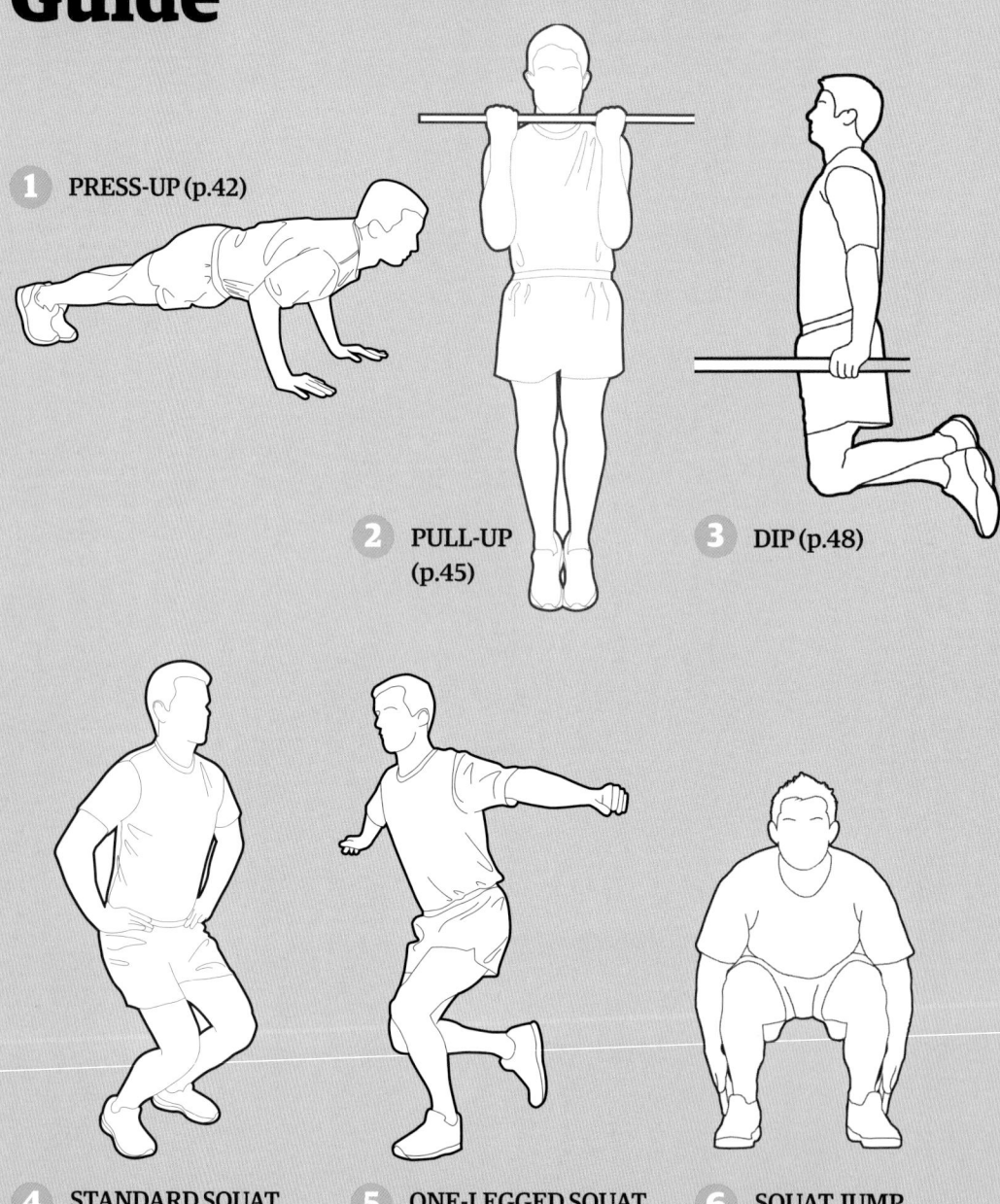

1 PRESS-UP (p.42)

2 PULL-UP (p.45)

3 DIP (p.48)

4 STANDARD SQUAT (p.50)

5 ONE-LEGGED SQUAT (p.51)

6 SQUAT JUMP (p.52)

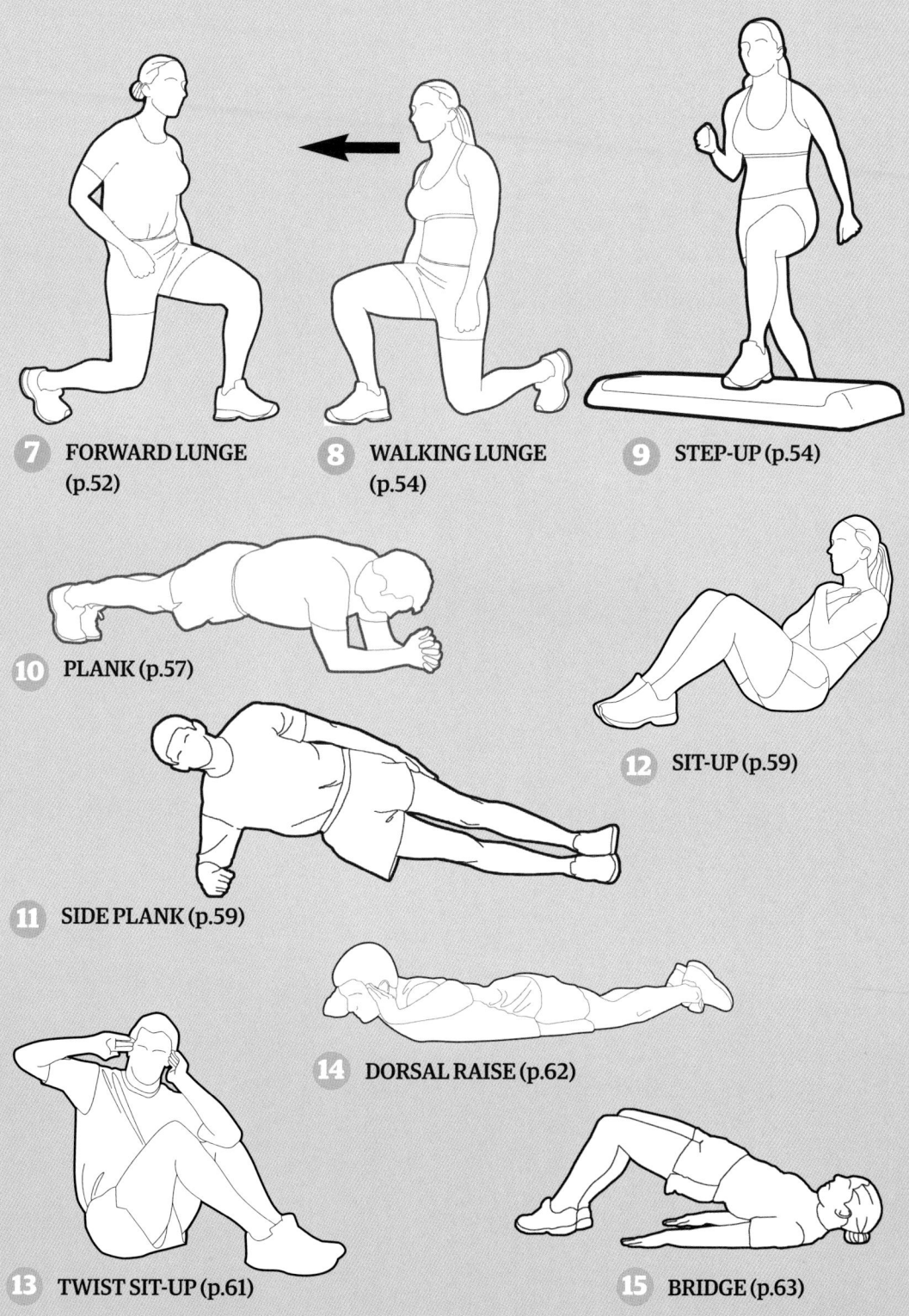

7 FORWARD LUNGE (p.52)

8 WALKING LUNGE (p.54)

9 STEP-UP (p.54)

10 PLANK (p.57)

12 SIT-UP (p.59)

11 SIDE PLANK (p.59)

14 DORSAL RAISE (p.62)

13 TWIST SIT-UP (p.61)

15 BRIDGE (p.63)

Exercise Programme Level One

	DAY 1	DAY 2
WEEK 1	**ASSESSMENT** ● Body mass index ● Waist-to-hip ratio ● Two-min press-up test ● Two-min sit-up test ● 2.4-km (1.5-mile) run test ● Sit-and-reach test	**STRENGTH** ● Warm-up ● 2 x 30 secs plank ● 2 x 10 secs bridge ● 2 x 10 twist sit-up ● 2 x 10 dorsal raise ● 2 x 10 forward lunge ● 2 x 10 standard squat **FLEXIBILITY** ● Stretch major muscles
WEEK 2	**AEROBIC** ● Warm-up ● Brisk walk for 10 mins; jog at 75% effort for 1 min when you feel ready ● 10-min cool-down and stretch	**STRENGTH** ● Warm-up ● 2 x 10 press-up ● 2 x 10 pull-up ● 2 x 10 dip ● 2 x 10 dorsal raise ● 2 x 10 sit-up **FLEXIBILITY** ● Stretch major muscles
WEEK 3	**AEROBIC** ● Warm-up ● Brisk walk for 15 mins; jog at 85% effort for 1 min when you feel ready ● 10-min cool-down and stretch	**STRENGTH** ● Warm-up ● 2 x 45 secs plank ● 2 x 12 secs bridge ● 2 x 12 twist sit-up ● 2 x 12 dorsal raise ● 2 x 12 forward lunge ● 2 x 12 standard squat **FLEXIBILITY** ● Stretch major muscles

REST DAY (between Day 1 and Day 2)

REST DAY (after Day 2)

DAY 3

DAY 4

AEROBIC
- Warm-up
- Jog for 5 mins out of a 10-min brisk walk
- 10-min cool-down and stretch

STRENGTH
- Warm-up
- 2 x 10 press-up
- 2 x 14 sit-up

FLEXIBILITY
- Stretch major muscles

REST DAY

AEROBIC
- Warm-up
- Jog for 10 mins out of a 15-min brisk walk
- 10-min cool-down and stretch

STRENGTH
- Warm-up
- 2 x 10 press-up
- 2 x 14 sit-up

FLEXIBILITY
- Stretch major muscles

REST DAY

AEROBIC
- Warm-up
- Jog for 12 mins out of a 20-min brisk walk
- 10-min cool-down and stretch

STRENGTH
- Warm-up
- 2 x 12 press-up
- 2 x 16 sit-up

FLEXIBILITY
- Stretch major muscles

REST DAY

	DAY 1	DAY 2
WEEK 4	**AEROBIC** ● Warm-up ● Brisk walk for 20 mins; jog at 70% effort for 2 mins when you feel ready ● 10-min cool-down and stretch	**STRENGTH** ● Warm-up ● 2 x 12 press-up ● 2 x 12 pull-up ● 2 x 12 dip ● 2 x 12 dorsal raise ● 2 x 12 sit-up **FLEXIBILITY** ● Stretch major muscles
WEEK 5	**AEROBIC** ● Warm-up ● Brisk walk for 25 mins; jog at 80% effort for 2 mins when you feel ready ● 10-min cool-down and stretch	**STRENGTH** ● Warm-up ● 2 x 60 secs plank ● 2 x 14 secs bridge ● 2 x 14 twist sit-up ● 2 x 14 dorsal raise ● 2 x 14 forward lunge ● 2 x 14 standard squat **FLEXIBILITY** ● Stretch major muscles
WEEK 6	**AEROBIC** ● Warm-up ● Brisk walk for 30 mins; jog at 85% effort for 2 mins when you feel ready ● 10-min cool-down and stretch	**STRENGTH** ● Warm-up ● 2 x 14 press-up ● 2 x 14 pull-up ● 2 x 14 dip ● 2 x 14 dorsal raise ● 2 x 14 sit-up **FLEXIBILITY** ● Stretch major muscles

REST DAY (Day 1) — REST DAY (Day 2)

DAY 3

DAY 4

AEROBIC
- Warm-up
- Jog for 15 mins out of a 25-min brisk walk
- 10-min cool-down and stretch

STRENGTH
- Warm-up
- 2 x 12 press-up
- 2 x 16 sit-up

FLEXIBILITY
- Stretch major muscles

REST DAY

AEROBIC
- Warm-up
- Jog for 20 mins out of a 30-min walk
- 10-min cool-down and stretch

STRENGTH
- Warm-up
- 2 x 14 press-up
- 2 x 18 sit-up

FLEXIBILITY
- Stretch major muscles

REST DAY

AEROBIC
- Warm-up
- Jog for 25 mins out of a 35-min brisk walk
- 10-min cool-down and stretch

ASSESSMENT
- Body mass index
- Waist-to-hip ratio
- Two-min press-up test
- Two-min sit-up test
- 2.4-km (1.5-mile) run test
- Sit-and-reach test

REST DAY

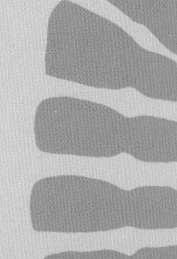

	DAY 1	DAY 2
WEEK 7	**AEROBIC** ● Warm-up ● 6 x 30 secs at 85% effort, 1 min recovery ● 10-min cool-down and stretch	**STRENGTH** ● Warm-up ● 3 x 30 secs bridge ● 3 x 10 twist sit-up ● 3 x 10 forward lunge ● 3 x 30 secs plank ● 3 x 10 dorsal raise ● 3 x 10 standard squat **FLEXIBILITY** ● Stretch major muscles
WEEK 8	**AEROBIC** ● Warm-up ● 4 x downhill reps at 85% effort, approx 150m each rep; walk uphill to recover ● 10-min cool-down and stretch	**STRENGTH** ● Warm-up ● 3 x 4–6 pull-up ● 3 x 10 dorsal raise ● 3 x 10 press-up ● 3 x 10 sit-up ● 3 x 10 dip **FLEXIBILITY** ● Stretch major muscles
WEEK 9	**AEROBIC** ● Warm-up ● 6 x 45 secs at 85% effort, 90 secs recovery ● 10-min cool-down and stretch	**STRENGTH** ● Warm-up ● 3 x 45 secs bridge ● 3 x 12 twist sit-up ● 3 x 12 forward lunge ● 3 x 45 secs plank ● 3 x 12 dorsal raise ● 3 x 12 standard squat **FLEXIBILITY** ● Stretch major muscles

REST DAY (after Day 1, each week)

REST DAY (after Day 2, each week)

DAY 3

AEROBIC & STRENGTH
● Warm-up
● 2 x 10 press-up
● 2 x 20 sit-up
● Jog for 30 mins (flat route) at 50–60% effort
● 10-min cool-down and stretch

STRENGTH CIRCUIT
● Warm-up
● 2 x 10 press-up
● 2 x 20 sit-up
● Jog for 30 mins (flat route) at 50–60% effort
● 3 x 50m sprints – 1 min rest
● 10-min cool-down and stretch

STRENGTH
● Warm-up
● 2 x 15 press-up
● 2 x 25 sit-up
● Jog for 35 mins (flat route) at 50–60% effort
● 4 x 50m sprints – 1 min rest
● 10-min cool-down and stretch

DAY 4

SPORT/CROSS TRAINING
● Warm-up
● 40 mins activity
● 10-min cool-down and stretch

REST DAY

SPORT/CROSS TRAINING
● Warm-up
● 40 mins activity
● 10-min cool-down and stretch

REST DAY

SPORT/CROSS TRAINING
● Warm-up
● 40 mins activity
● 10-min cool-down and stretch

REST DAY

	DAY 1	**DAY 2**

WEEK 10

DAY 1

AEROBIC
- Warm-up
- 4 x uphill reps at 85% effort, approx 150m each rep; walk downhill to recover
- 10-min cool-down and stretch

DAY 2

STRENGTH CIRCUIT
- Warm-up
- 3 x 6–8 pull-up
- 3 x 12 dorsal raise
- 3 x 12 press-up
- 3 x 12 sit-up
- 3 x 12 chair dip

FLEXIBILITY
- Stretch major muscles

REST DAY

REST DAY

WEEK 11

DAY 1

AEROBIC
- Warm-up
- 6 x 1 min at 85% effort, 2-min recovery
- 10-min cool-down and stretch

DAY 2

STRENGTH CIRCUIT
- Warm-up
- 3 x 60 secs bridge
- 3 x 15 twist sit-up
- 3 x 15 forward lunge
- 3 x 60 secs plank
- 3 x 15 dorsal raise
- 3 x 15 standard squat

FLEXIBILITY
- Stretch major muscles

REST DAY

REST DAY

WEEK 12

DAY 1

AEROBIC
- Warm-up
- 4 x downhill reps at 85% effort, approx 150m each rep; walk uphill to recover
- 10-min cool-down and stretch

DAY 2

STRENGTH CIRCUIT
- Warm-up
- 3 x 10 pull-up
- 3 x 15 dorsal raise
- 3 x 15 press-up
- 3 x 15 dip
- 3 x 15 sit-up

FLEXIBILITY
- Stretch major muscles

REST DAY

REST DAY

DAY 3

DAY 4

AEROBIC & STRENGTH
- Warm-up
- 3 x 12 press-up
- 3 x 20 sit-up
- Jog for 40 mins (flat route) at 50–60% effort
- 5 x 50m sprints – 1 min rest
- 10-min cool-down and stretch

SPORT/CROSS TRAINING
- Warm-up
- 40 mins activity
- 10-min cool-down and stretch

REST DAY

AEROBIC & STRENGTH
- Warm-up
- 3 x 15 press-up
- 3 x 20 sit-up
- Jog for 45 mins (flat route) at 50–60% effort
- 5 x 50m sprints – 1 min rest
- 10-min cool-down and stretch

SPORT/CROSS TRAINING
- Warm-up
- 40 mins activity
- 10-min cool-down and stretch

REST DAY

AEROBIC
- Warm-up
- Jog for 20 mins (flat route) at 50–60% effort
- 5-min cool-down and stretch

FLEXIBILITY
- Stretch major muscles

ASSESSMENT
- Body mass index
- Waist-to-hip ratio
- Two-min press-up test
- Two-min sit-up test
- 2.4-km (1.5-mile) run test
- Sit-and-reach test

REST DAY

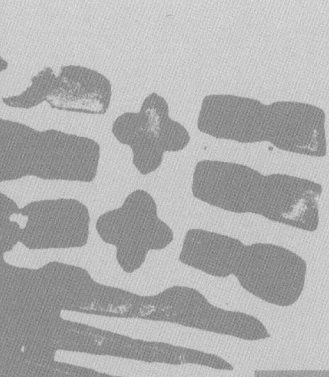

Exercise Programme Level Two

	DAY 1	DAY 2
WEEK 1	**ASSESSMENT** ● Body mass index ● Waist-to-hip ratio ● Two-min press-up test ● Two-min sit-up test ● 2.4-km (1.5-mile) run test ● Sit-and-reach test	**STRENGTH CIRCUIT** ● Warm-up ● 3 x 45 secs plank ● 3 x 20 dorsal raise ● 3 x 8 walking lunge ● 3 x 45 secs bridge ● 3 x 10 crunch ● 3 x 8 standard squat (1 sec hold) **FLEXIBILITY** ● Stretch major muscles
WEEK 2	**AEROBIC** ● Warm-up ● 10-min jog ● 6 x 90 secs at 85% effort, 3-min slow walk to recover ● 10-min cool-down and stretch	**STRENGTH CIRCUIT** ● Warm-up ● 3 x 6–8 pull-up ● 3 x 20 press-up ● 3 x 20 dorsal raise ● 3 x 20 dip ● 3 x 20 sit-up **FLEXIBILITY** ● Stretch major muscles
WEEK 3	**AEROBIC** ● Warm-up ● 10-min jog ● 5 x uphill reps at 90% effort, approx 150m each rep; walk downhill to recover ● 10-min cool-down and stretch	**STRENGTH CIRCUIT** ● Warm-up ● 3 x 60 secs plank ● 3 x 20 dorsal raise ● 3 x 10 walking lunge ● 3 x 60 secs bridge ● 3 x 12 crunch ● 3 x 10 standard squat (1 sec hold) **FLEXIBILITY** ● Stretch major muscles

REST DAY (between Day 1 and Day 2)

REST DAY (after Day 2)

DAY 3

DAY 4

AEROBIC & STRENGTH
- Warm-up
- 3 x 20 press-up
- 3 x 25 sit-up
- Steady state run 40 mins (flat route) at 60-70% effort
- 3 x 150m sprints at 80-90% effort with equal distance walk between each one
- 10-min cool-down and stretch

SPORT/CROSS TRAINING
- Warm-up
- 40 mins activity
- 10-min cool-down and stretch

REST DAY

AEROBIC & STRENGTH
- Warm-up
- Steady state run 40 mins (undulating route) at 60-70% effort
- 3 x 20 press-up
- 3 x 25 sit-up
- 3 x 150m sprints at 80-90% effort with equal distance walk between each one
- 10-min cool-down and stretch

SPORT/CROSS TRAINING
- Warm-up
- 40 mins activity
- 10-min cool-down and stretch

REST DAY

AEROBIC & STRENGTH
- Warm-up
- 4 x 18 press-up
- 4 x 20 sit-up
- Steady state run 45 mins (flat route) at 60-70% effort
- 4 x 150m sprints at 80-90% effort with equal distance walk between each one
- 10-min cool-down and stretch

SPORT/CROSS TRAINING
- Warm-up
- 50 mins activity
- 10-min cool-down and stretch

REST DAY

	DAY 1	**DAY 2**
WEEK 4	**AEROBIC** ● Warm-up ● 10-min jog ● 6 x 90 secs at 85% effort, 3-min slow walk to recover ● 10-min cool-down and stretch	**STRENGTH CIRCUIT** ● Warm-up ● 3 x 8-10 pull-up ● 3 x 18 press-up ● 3 x 25 dorsal raise ● 3 x 25 dip ● 3 x 25 sit-up **FLEXIBILITY** ● Stretch major muscles
WEEK 5	**AEROBIC** ● Warm-up ● 10-min jog ● 5 x downhill reps at 90% effort, approx 150m each rep; walk uphill to recover ● 10-min cool-down and stretch	**STRENGTH CIRCUIT** ● Warm-up ● 3 x 60 secs plank ● 3 x 20 dorsal raise ● 3 x 10 walking lunge ● 3 x 60 secs bridge ● 3 x 12 crunch ● 3 x 10 standard squat (1 sec hold) **FLEXIBILITY** ● Stretch major muscles
WEEK 6	**AEROBIC** ● Warm-up ● 10-min jog ● 6 x 90 secs at 85% effort, 3-min slow walk to recover ● 10-min cool-down and stretch	**STRENGTH CIRCUIT** ● 3 x 8 pull-up ● 3 x 20 press-up ● 3 x 20 dorsal raise ● 3 x 25 dip ● 3 x 20 sit-up **FLEXIBILITY** ● Stretch major muscles

REST DAY REST DAY

REST DAY REST DAY

REST DAY REST DAY

DAY 3

DAY 4

AEROBIC & STRENGTH
- Warm-up
- Steady state run 45 mins (undulating route) at 60-70% effort
- 4 x 18 press-up
- 4 x 20 sit-up
- 4 x 150m sprints at 80-90% effort with equal distance walk between each one
- 10-min cool-down and stretch

SPORT/CROSS TRAINING
- Warm-up
- 50 mins activity
- 10-min cool-down and stretch

REST DAY

AEROBIC & STRENGTH
- Warm-up
- 4 x 20 press-up
- 4 x 20 sit-up
- Steady state run 45 mins (flat route) at 60-70% effort
- 5 x 150m sprints at 80-90% effort with equal distance walk between each one
- 10-min cool-down and stretch

SPORT/CROSS TRAINING
- Warm-up
- 60 mins activity
- 10-min cool-down and stretch

REST DAY

AEROBIC
- Warm-up
- Steady state run 30 mins (undulating route) at 60-70% effort
- 6 x 150m sprints at 80-90% effort with equal distance walk between each one
- 10-min cool-down and stretch

ASSESSMENT
- Body mass index
- Waist-to-hip ratio
- Two-min press-up test
- Two-min sit-up test
- 2.4-km (1.5-mile) run test
- Sit-and-reach test

REST DAY

	DAY 1	**DAY 2**	
WEEK 7	**AEROBIC** ● Warm-up ● 10-min jog ● 5 x uphill reps at 90% effort, approx 200m each rep; walk downhill to recover ● 10-min cool-down and stretch	**STRENGTH CIRCUIT** ● Warm-up ● 4 x 45 secs plank ● 4 x 20 dorsal raise ● 4 x 12 walking lunge ● 4 x 45 secs bridge ● 4 x 14 crunch ● 4 x 12 standard squat (1 sec hold) **FLEXIBILITY** ● Stretch major muscles	
WEEK 8	**AEROBIC** ● Warm-up ● 10-min jog ● 6 x 90 secs at 85% effort, 3-min slow walk to recover ● 10-min cool-down and stretch	**STRENGTH CIRCUIT** ● Warm-up ● 4 x 8 pull-up ● 4 x 20 press-up ● 4 x 20 dorsal raise ● 4 x 25 dip ● 4 x 20 sit-up **FLEXIBILITY** ● Stretch major muscles	
WEEK 9	**AEROBIC** ● Warm-up ● 10-min jog ● 5 x uphill reps at 90% effort, approx 200m each rep; walk downhill to recover ● 10-min cool-down and stretch	**STRENGTH CIRCUIT** ● Warm-up ● 4 x 45 secs plank ● 4 x 20 dorsal raise ● 4 x 12 walking lunge ● 4 x 45 secs bridge ● 4 x 14 crunch ● 4 x 12 standard squat (1 sec hold) **FLEXIBILITY** ● Stretch major muscles	

REST DAY (between Day 1 and Day 2, and after Day 2) for each week.

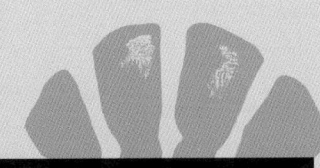

DAY 3

DAY 4

AEROBIC & STRENGTH
- Warm-up
- 4 x 20 press-up
- 4 x 25 sit-up
- Steady state run 50 mins (flat route) at 60-70% effort
- 3 x 200m sprints at 80-90% effort with equal distance walk between each one
- 10-min cool-down and stretch

SPORT/CROSS TRAINING
- Warm-up
- 60 mins activity
- 10-min cool-down and stretch

REST DAY

AEROBIC & STRENGTH
- Warm-up
- 4 x 25 press-up
- 4 x 30 sit-up
- Steady state run 50 mins (flat route) at 60-70% effort
- 5 x 200m sprints at 80-90% effort with equal distance walk between each one
- 10-min cool-down and stretch

SPORT/CROSS TRAINING
- Warm-up
- 60 mins activity
- 10-min cool-down and stretch

REST DAY

AEROBIC & STRENGTH
- Warm-up
- 2 x 15 press-up
- 2 x 25 sit-up
- Jog for 35 mins (flat route)
- 4 x 50m sprints - 1 min rest
- 10-min cool-down and stretch

SPORT/CROSS TRAINING
- Warm-up
- 60 mins activity
- 10-min cool-down and stretch

REST DAY

	DAY 1	DAY 2	

WEEK 10

DAY 1

AEROBIC
- Warm-up
- 10-min jog
- 6 x 90 secs at 85% effort, 3-min slow walk to recover
- 10-min cool-down and stretch

REST DAY

DAY 2

STRENGTH CIRCUIT
- Warm-up
- 4 x 8-10 pull-up
- 4 x 25 press-up
- 4 x 20 dip
- 4 x 15 dorsal raise
- 4 x 25 sit-up

FLEXIBILITY
- Stretch major muscles

REST DAY

WEEK 11

AEROBIC
- Warm-up
- 10-min jog
- 5 x downhill reps at 90% effort, approx 200m each rep; walk uphill to recover
- 10-min cool-down and stretch

REST DAY

STRENGTH CIRCUIT
- 4 x 60 secs plank
- 4 x 20 dorsal raise
- 4 x 12 walking lunge
- 4 x 60 secs bridge
- 4 x 15 crunch
- 4 x 14 standard squat (1 sec hold)

FLEXIBILITY
- Stretch major muscles

REST DAY

WEEK 12

AEROBIC
- Warm-up
- 10-min jog
- 6 x 90 secs at 85% effort, 3-min slow walk to recover
- 10-min cool-down and stretch

REST DAY

STRENGTH CIRCUIT
- Warm-up
- 4 x 10 pull-up
- 4 x 25 press-up
- 4 x 20 dip
- 4 x 15 dorsal raise

FLEXIBILITY
- Stretch major muscles

REST DAY

DAY 3

DAY 4

AEROBIC & STRENGTH
- Warm-up
- Steady state run 50 mins (undulating route) at 60-70% effort
- 4 x 25 press-up
- 4 x 30 sit-up
- 6 x 200m sprints at 80-90% effort with equal distance walk between each one
- 10-min cool-down and stretch

SPORT/CROSS TRAINING
- Warm-up
- 60 mins activity
- 10-min cool-down and stretch

REST DAY

AEROBIC & STRENGTH
- Warm-up
- 4 x 25 press-up
- 4 x 30 sit-up
- Steady state run 35 mins (flat route) at 60-70% effort
- 6 x 200m sprints at 80-90% effort, equal distance walk between each one
- 10-min cool-down and stretch

SPORT/CROSS TRAINING
- Warm-up
- 40 mins activity
- 10-min cool-down and stretch

REST DAY

AEROBIC & STRENGTH
- Warm-up
- Steady state run 40 mins (flat route) at 60-70% effort
- 10-min cool-down and stretch

ASSESSMENT
- Body mass index
- Waist-to-hip ratio
- Two-min press-up test
- Two-min sit-up test
- 2.4-km (1.5-mile) run test
- Sit-and-reach test

REST DAY

139

Exercise Programme Level Three

	DAY 1	DAY 2

WEEK 1

DAY 1

ASSESSMENT
- Body mass index
- Waist-to-hip ratio
- Two-min press-up test
- Two-min sit-up test
- 2.4-km (1.5-mile) run test
- Sit-and-reach test

REST DAY

DAY 2

STRENGTH
- Warm-up
- 3 x 60 secs plank
- 3 x 15 dorsal raise
- 3 x 6 squat jump
- 3 x 15 secs bridge leg extension (each leg)
- 3 x 15 crunch
- 3 x 6 backward lunge
- 3 x 30 side plank (each side)
- 3 x 8 one-legged squat (4 each leg)

FLEXIBILITY
- Stretch major muscles

REST DAY

WEEK 2

DAY 1

AEROBIC
- Warm-up
- 10-min jog
- 6 x 2 mins at 85% effort, 3-min slow walk to recover
- 10-min cool-down and stretch

REST DAY

DAY 2

STRENGTH
- Warm-up
- 3 x 8 overhand pull-up
- 3 x 10 wide-arm press-up
- 3 x 10 half-sit
- 3 x 10 dip
- 3 x 10 close-arm press-up
- 3 x 10 crunch
- 3 x 8 pull-up
- 3 x 10 sit-up

FLEXIBILITY
- Stretch major muscles

REST DAY

WEEK 3

DAY 1

AEROBIC
- Warm-up
- 10-min jog
- 5 x uphill reps at 90% effort, approx 200m each rep; walk downhill to recover
- 10-min cool-down and stretch

REST DAY

DAY 2

STRENGTH
- Warm-up
- 3 x 60 secs plank
- 3 x 15 dorsal raise
- 3 x 8 squat jump
- 3 x 20 secs bridge leg extension (each leg)
- 3 x 15 crunch
- 3 x 8 backward lunge
- 3 x 45 secs side plank (each side)
- 3 x 10 one-legged squat (5 each leg)

FLEXIBILITY
- Stretch major muscles

REST DAY

DAY 3

AEROBIC & STRENGTH
- Warm-up
- 2 x 1-min press-up
- 2 x 1-min sit-up
- Steady state run 50 mins (flat route) at 60-70% effort
- 3 x 250m sprints at 80-90% effort with equal distance walk between each one
- 10-min cool-down and stretch

AEROBIC & STRENGTH
- Warm-up
- Steady state run 50 mins (undulating route) at 60-70% effort
- 2 x 1-min press-up
- 2 x 1-min sit-up
- 3 x 250m sprints at 80-90% effort with equal distance walk between each one
- 10-min cool-down and stretch

AEROBIC & STRENGTH
- Warm-up
- 2 x 1-min press-up
- 2 x 1-min sit-up
- Steady state run 50 mins (flat route) at 60-70% effort
- 4 x 250m sprints at 80-90% effort with equal distance walk between each one
- 10-min cool-down and stretch

DAY 4

SPORT/CROSS TRAINING
- Warm-up
- 60 mins activity

FLEXIBILITY
- Stretch major muscles

REST DAY

SPORT/CROSS TRAINING
- Warm-up
- 60 mins activity

FLEXIBILITY
- Stretch major muscles

REST DAY

SPORT/CROSS TRAINING
- Warm-up
- 60 mins activity

FLEXIBILITY
- Stretch major muscles

REST DAY

141

	DAY 1	DAY 2
WEEK 4	**AEROBIC** ● Warm-up ● 10-min jog ● 6 x 90 secs at 85% effort, 3-min slow walk to recover ● 10-min cool-down and stretch	**STRENGTH** ● Warm-up ● 3 x 8 overhand pull-up ● 3 x 12 wide-arm press-up ● 3 x 12 half sit ● 3 x 12 dip ● 3 x 12 close-arm press-up ● 3 x 12 crunch ● 3 x 8 pull-up ● 3 x 12 sit-up **FLEXIBILITY** ● Stretch major muscles
WEEK 5	**AEROBIC** ● Warm-up ● 10-min jog ● 5 x downhill reps at 90% effort, approx 200m each rep; walk uphill to recover ● 10-min cool-down and stretch	**STRENGTH** ● Warm-up ● 3 x 60 secs plank ● 3 x 15 dorsal raise ● 3 x 10 squat jump ● 3 x 30 secs bridge leg extension (each leg) ● 3 x 15 crunch ● 3 x 10 backward lunge ● 3 x 60 secs side plank (each side) ● 3 x 10 single-leg squat **FLEXIBILITY** ● Stretch major muscles
WEEK 6	**AEROBIC** ● Warm-up ● 10-min jog ● 6 x 90 secs at 85% effort, 3-min slow walk to recover ● 10-min cool-down and stretch	**STRENGTH** ● 3 x 10 overhand pull-up ● 3 x 15 wide-arm press-up ● 3 x 15 half sit ● 3 x 15 dip ● 3 x 15 close-arm press-up ● 3 x 15 crunch ● 3 x 10 pull-up ● 3 x 15 sit-up **FLEXIBILITY** ● Stretch major muscles

REST DAY

REST DAY

DAY 3

DAY 4

AEROBIC & STRENGTH
- Warm-up
- Steady state run 50 min (undulating route) at 60–70% effort
- 2 x 1-min press-up
- 2 x 1-min sit-up
- 4 x 250m sprints at 80–90% effort with equal distance walk between each one
- 10-min cool-down and stretch

SPORT/CROSS TRAINING
- Warm-up
- 60 mins activity

FLEXIBILITY
- Stretch major muscles

REST DAY

AEROBIC & STRENGTH
- Warm-up
- 2 x 1-min press-up
- 2 x 1-min press-up
- Steady state run 50 mins (flat route) at 60–70% effort
- 5 x 250m sprints at 80–90% effort with equal distance walk between each one
- 10-min cool-down and stretch

SPORT/CROSS TRAINING
- Warm-up
- 60 mins activity

FLEXIBILITY
- Stretch major muscles

REST DAY

AEROBIC
- Warm-up
- Steady state run 50 mins (undulating route) at 60–70% effort
- 10-min cool-down and stretch

ASSESSMENT
- Body mass index
- Waist-to-hip ratio
- Two-min press-up test
- Two-min sit-up test
- 2.4-km (1.5-mile) run test
- Sit-and-reach test

REST DAY

143

	DAY 1	**DAY 2**

WEEK 7

DAY 1

AEROBIC
- Warm-up
- 10-min jog
- 5 x uphill reps at 90% effort, approx 200m each rep; walk downhill to recover
- 10-min cool-down and stretch

DAY 2

STRENGTH
- Warm-up
- 3 x 60 secs plank
- 3 x 15 dorsal raise
- 3 x 10 squat jump
- 3 x 10 step-up (each leg)
- 3 x 45 secs bridge leg extension (each leg)
- 3 x 15 crunch
- 3 x 10 walking lunge (each leg)
- 3 x 90 secs side plank (each side)
- 3 x 10 single-leg squat

FLEXIBILITY
- Stretch major muscles

REST DAY — REST DAY

WEEK 8

DAY 1

AEROBIC
- Warm-up
- 10-min jog
- 6 x 90 secs at 85% effort, 3-min slow walk to recover
- 10-min cool-down and stretch

DAY 2

STRENGTH
- Warm-up
- 4 x 12 overhand pull-up
- 4 x 10 wide-arm press-up
- 4 x 10 half sit
- 4 x 20 dip
- 4 x 10 close-arm press-up
- 4 x 10 crunch
- 4 x 12 pull-up
- 4 x 10 sit-up

FLEXIBILITY
- Stretch major muscles

REST DAY — REST DAY

WEEK 9

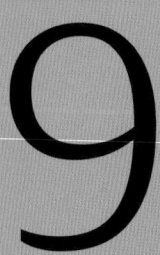

DAY 1

AEROBIC
- Warm-up
- 10-min jog
- 5 x uphill reps at 90% effort, approx 200m each rep; walk downhill to recover
- 10-min cool-down and stretch

DAY 2

STRENGTH
- Warm-up
- 3 x 60 secs plank
- 3 x 15 dorsal raise
- 3 x 10 squat jump
- 3 x 8 step-up (each leg)
- 3 x 45 secs bridge leg extension (each leg)
- 3 x 15 crunch
- 3 x 8 walking lunge (each leg)
- 3 x 60 secs side plank (each side)
- 3 x 12 one-legged squat

FLEXIBILITY
- Stretch major muscles

REST DAY — REST DAY

DAY 3

DAY 4

AEROBIC & STRENGTH
- Warm-up
- 2 x 90 secs press-up
- 2 x 90 secs sit-up
- Steady state run 50 mins (undulating route) at 60-70% effort
- 5 x 250m sprints at 80-90% effort with equal distance walk between each one
- 10-min cool-down and stretch

SPORT/CROSS TRAINING
- Warm-up
- 60 mins activity

FLEXIBILITY
- Stretch major muscles

REST DAY

AEROBIC & STRENGTH
- Warm-up
- Steady state run 50 mins (flat route) at 60-70% effort
- 2 x 90 secs press-up
- 2 x 90 secs sit-up
- 6 x 250m sprints at 80-90% effort with equal distance walk between each one
- 10-min cool-down and stretch

SPORT/CROSS TRAINING
- Warm-up
- 60 mins activity

FLEXIBILITY
- Stretch major muscles

REST DAY

AEROBIC & STRENGTH
- Warm-up
- 2 x 90 secs press-up
- 2 x 90 secs sit-up
- Steady state run 50 mins (undulating route) at 60-70% effort
- 6 x 250m sprints at 80-90% effort with equal distance walk between each one
- 10-min cool-down and stretch

SPORT/CROSS TRAINING
- Warm-up
- 60 mins activity

FLEXIBILITY
- Stretch major muscles

REST DAY

	DAY 1	**DAY 2**

WEEK 10

DAY 1

AEROBIC
- Warm-up
- 10-min jog
- 6 x 90 secs at 85% effort, 3-min slow walk to recover
- 10-min cool-down and stretch

REST DAY

DAY 2

STRENGTH
- Warm-up
- 4 x 12 overhand pull-up
- 4 x 10 wide-arm press-up
- 4 x 10 half-sit
- 4 x 20 dip
- 4 x 10 close-arm press-up
- 4 x 10 crunch
- 4 x 12 pull-up
- 4 x 10 sit-up

FLEXIBILITY
- Stretch major muscles

REST DAY

WEEK 11

AEROBIC
- Warm-up
- 10-min jog
- 5 x downhill reps at 90% effort, approx 250m each rep; walk uphill to recover
- 10-min cool-down and stretch

REST DAY

STRENGTH
- Warm-up
- 3 x 60 secs plank
- 3 x 15 dorsal raise
- 3 x 10 squat jump
- 3 x 10 step-up (each leg)
- 3 x 30 secs bridge leg extension
- 3 x 15 crunch
- 3 x 10 walking lunge (each leg)
- 3 x 60 secs side plank (each side)
- 3 x 10 single-leg squat

FLEXIBILITY
- Stretch major muscles

REST DAY

WEEK 12

AEROBIC
- Warm-up
- 10-min jog
- 6 x 90 secs at 85% effort, 3-min slow walk to recover
- 10-min cool-down and stretch

REST DAY

STRENGTH
- Warm-up
- 3 x 12 overhand pull-up
- 3 x 10 wide-arm press-up
- 3 x 10 half-sit
- 3 x 20 dip
- 3 x 10 close-arm press-up
- 3 x 10 crunch
- 3 x 12 pull-up
- 3 x 10 sit-up

FLEXIBILITY
- Stretch major muscles

REST DAY

DAY 3

AEROBIC & STRENGTH
- Warm-up
- Steady state run 50 mins (flat route) at 60–70% effort
- 2 x 90 secs press-up
- 2 x 90 secs sit-up
- 6 x 250m sprints at 80–90% effort with equal distance walk between each one
- 10-min cool-down and stretch

AEROBIC & STRENGTH
- Warm-up
- 2 x 90 secs press-up
- 2 x 90 secs sit-up
- Steady state run 50 mins (undulating route) at 60–70% effort
- 6 x 250m sprints at 80–90% effort with equal distance walk between each one
- 10-min cool-down and stretch

AEROBIC
- Warm-up
- Steady state run 40 mins (flat route) at 60–70% effort
- 10-min cool-down and stretch

DAY 4

SPORT/CROSS TRAINING
- Warm-up
- 60 mins activity

FLEXIBILITY
- Stretch major muscles

REST DAY

SPORT/CROSS TRAINING
- Warm-up
- 60 mins activity

FLEXIBILITY
- Stretch major muscles

REST DAY

ASSESSMENT
- Body mass index
- Waist-to-hip ratio
- Two-min press-up test
- Two-min sit-up test
- 2.4-km (1.5-mile) run test
- Sit-and-reach test

REST DAY

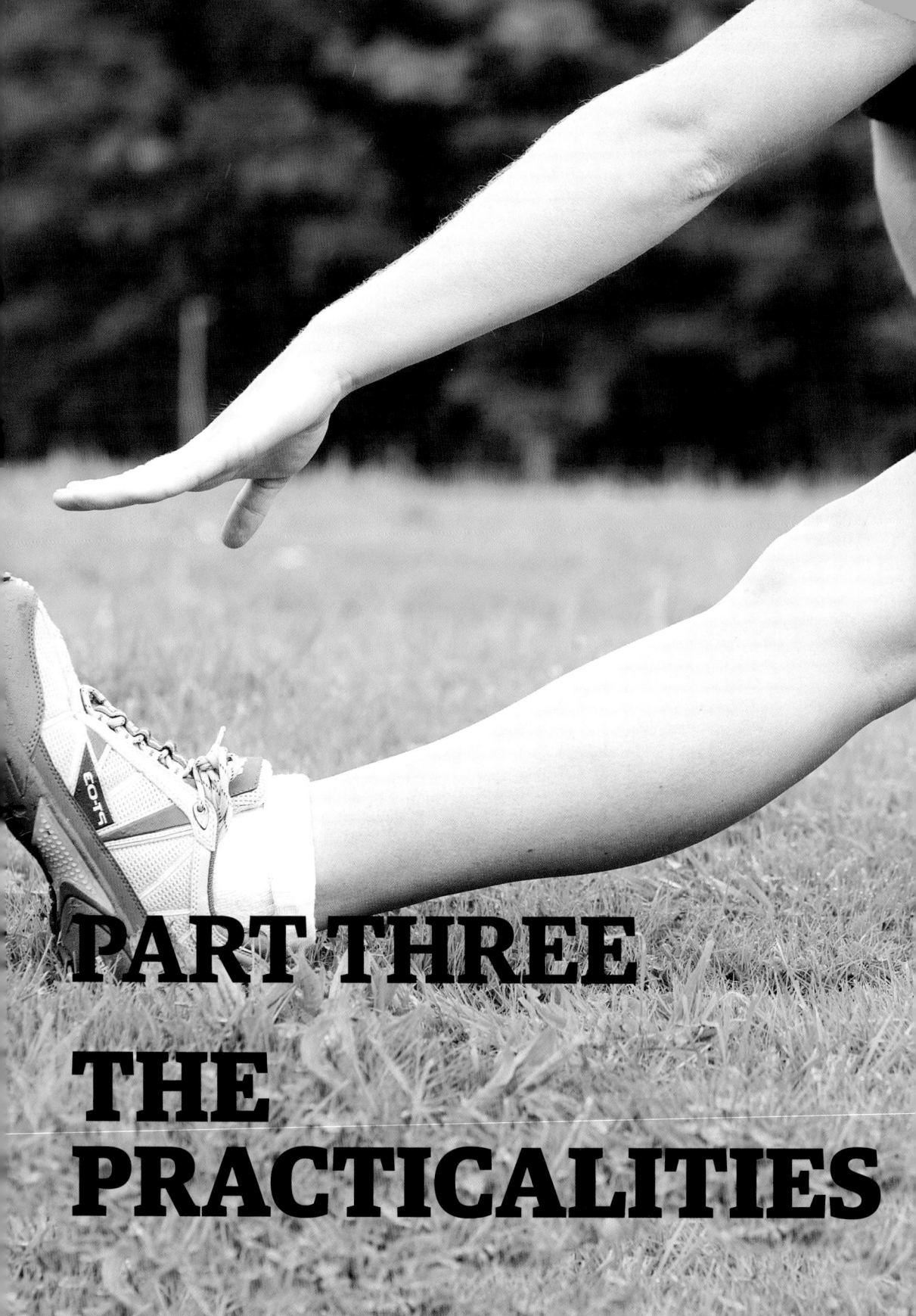

PART THREE
THE
PRACTICALITIES

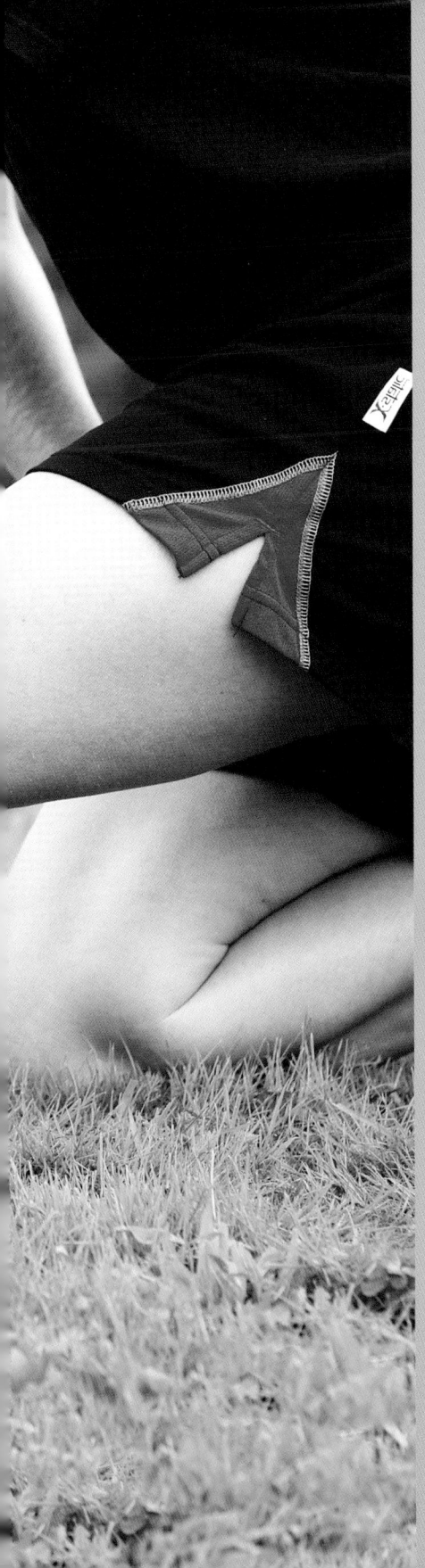

This part of the book is all about the practicalities of getting and staying fit. In other words, it shows you how to put the principles you've learned into practice in the safest and most effective way.

That entails everything from lifting weights correctly to identifying the early signs of possible injury or illness, and staying safe when you're exercising outdoors.

There is also advice on fuelling your workouts with the right nutrition and hydration strategies, information on how to select the right shoes for your sport, what to wear for workouts and the equipment and gadgets that can help you monitor your progress and get the most out of each session. Since regular, consistent exercise is the key to success, the final chapter addresses motivation and how to stick with the programme when the going gets tough.

Staying healthy

As any athlete knows, consistency is key to improving fitness performance. So there is nothing worse than being hampered by injury. Sensible preventative procedures, such as beginning a session with a warm-up, ending with a cool-down and progressing at an appropriate rate, will help minimise the risks. But there are a few other precautions worth taking to avoid both chronic (overuse) and acute (sudden onset) injuries.

Be body aware

Always use good technique when you are warming up, exercising and stretching. Do not use momentum or force to put yourself into a position or lift a weight that you cannot achieve with control. It can help to use a mirror to check your form and posture during workouts.

Lift weights safely

Whether it is a heavy box or a dumbbell, there are a few rules that you should observe when lifting any weight from the floor:

Stand close to the object, with feet hip-distance apart and knees bent.

Take hold of the item and bring it close to your body before pushing up through the feet to standing.

NEVER bend forwards from the waist as this can potentially damage your back.

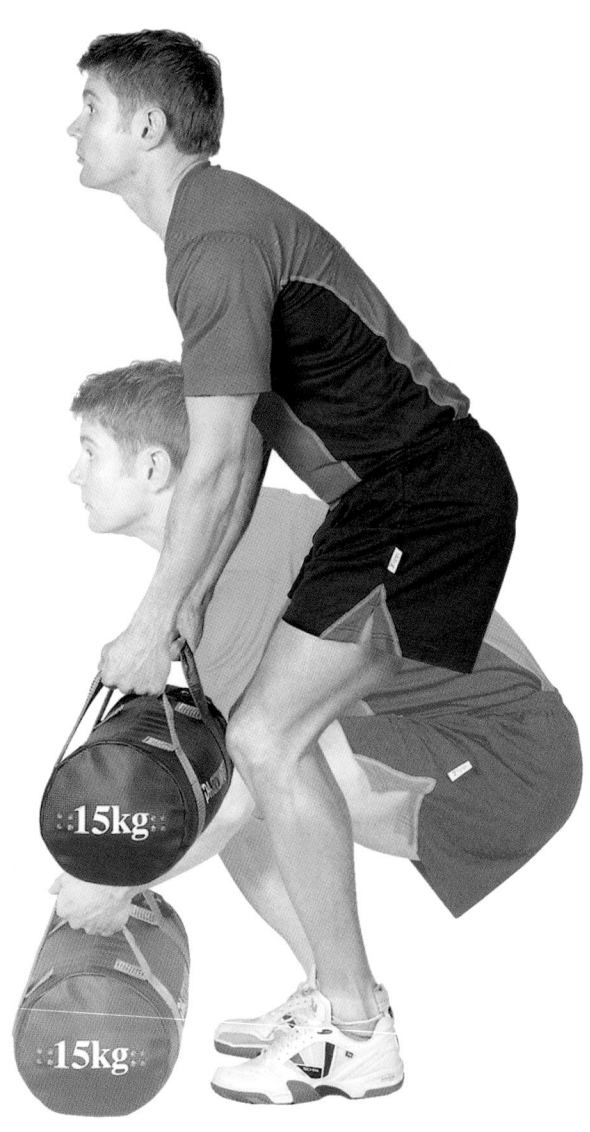

Run safely

Running gets a bad name in the injury stakes - as many as 7 out of 10 runners are halted by injury in any given year. While poor technique is often to blame, people also attempt to do too much, too soon. The Army has identified a strong relation between aerobic fitness and risk of injury – slow runners are three times more likely to get injured than fast runners during basic training.

If you are unlucky enough to sustain a musculoskeletal injury, such as a strain or sprain, act immediately. The quicker you address the problem, the more you can limit the extent of the damage. If the injury is severe, seek medical help straightaway. For less serious problems, such as a muscle pull, apply the RICE strategy.

The acronym RICE stands for Rest, Ice, Compression and Elevation.

REST Immobilise the injured part of the body and take weight off the injured limb or area.

ICE Apply ice, in the form of an ice pack or bag of frozen peas, for eight minutes every three hours.

Ten ways to run away from injury

- Don't run every day. Mix running with low-impact activities such as swimming, cycling and rowing.
- Alternate hard sessions with easier ones.
- Warm up properly, cool down and stretch each time you run.
- Don't try to progress too quickly – allow your body to adapt to the new challenge being placed upon it.
- Wear the right footwear for your individual needs and the surfaces you are running on.
- Try to get a mix of surfaces, rather than always running on tarmac or concrete.
- Build up the strength in your muscles, tendons, ligaments and bones through strength training.
- Stay well hydrated.
- Only increase your mileage/running time by 5-10% each week.
- Don't ignore aches and pains. Running through pain can cause a full-blown injury.

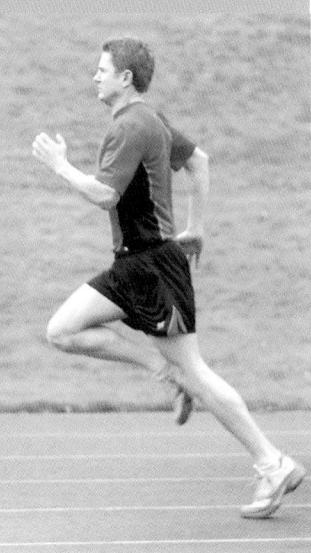

COMPRESSION Apply a compression bandage to the area to limit blood flow and reduce swelling.

ELEVATION Elevate the area, if possible, so that blood flows away from the injury. For example, raise your leg above hip height.

Continue with the RICE measures for 48 hours. After that, you need to start mobilising and stretching the injured area. If you are not able to do this, or if it is too painful to do so, seek advice from a sports medicine expert or doctor.

Common injuries

Here are some of the most common injuries you may encounter as a result of physical training, and steps you can take to prevent them happening:

ILIOTIBIAL BAND (ITB) SYNDROME

The ITB is a band of connective tissue that stretches from the hip to just below the knee, along the side of the thigh. It can become overtight and inflamed, causing it to pull on or rub against other surrounding tissues.

PREVENT BY...

strengthening the glutes (see the exercises on pp.50-55), avoiding too much downhill running or cambered surfaces, correcting overpronation (this is when the foot rolls in too quickly or too much on landing).

HAMSTRING TEARS

Muscle tears in this area result from excessive strain on the muscle, either as a result of a sudden movement, or a repeated pattern of movement (an "overuse" injury).

PREVENT BY...

warming up thoroughly, working on your technique, stretching and not building up your training too quickly.

ACHILLES TENDONITIS

This is inflammation of the Achilles tendon along the back of the lower leg. You may feel stiff and tender at the back of the heel, particularly in the morning and when rising up on to your toes.

PREVENT BY...

stretching your calves, wearing the right running shoes, performing calf raises (p.68).

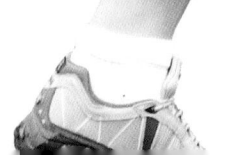

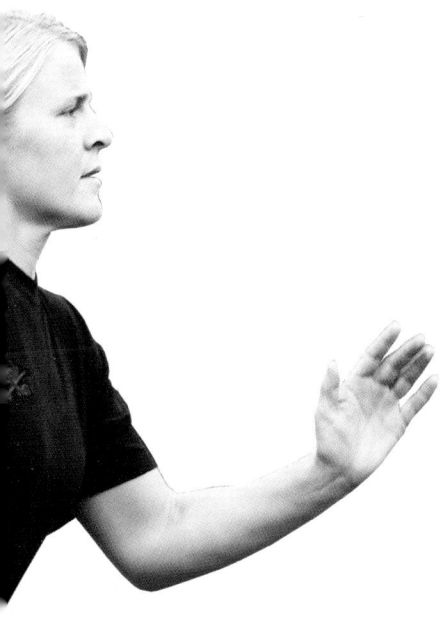

KNEE PAIN

Patellofemoral syndrome, or "runner's knee" is often a result of the kneecap maltracking, causing inflammation and pain beneath it.

PREVENT BY...

strengthening the thighs by doing squats, lunges and step-ups, stretching regularly, wearing appropriate running shoes.

SHIN SPLINTS

This term broadly describes inflammation of the connective tissue that attaches to the main shinbone, the tibia. It causes a general tenderness or bruised feeling.

PREVENT BY...

changing your shoes regularly, not running on hard surfaces all the time, stretching and strengthening the lower legs.

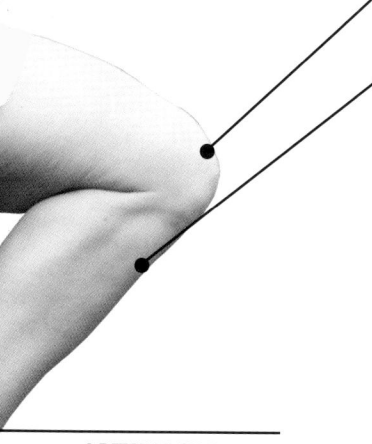

ANKLE SPRAIN

"Turning" your ankle may just result in a slight stretch of the ligaments while a full-blown sprain will actually tear the tissues, causing swelling and bruising.

PREVENT BY...

watching your step, particularly on uneven ground, strengthening your ankles using single-leg balance exercises or a wobble board (an unstable disc on which you stand and attempt to stay balanced).

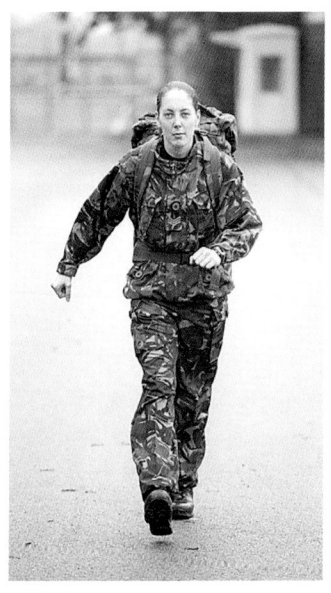

Cross training

Even if an injury does put you out of action for a couple of weeks or more, there is no need to go back to square one with your fitness. "Cross training" should enable you to maintain your fitness while the injury heals. Cross training basically means choosing activities that allow you to take the injured part of your body out of the equation. For example, you may not be able to run, but you could swim. Non-weight bearing or low-impact exercise is usually the best choice.

PTI Tip

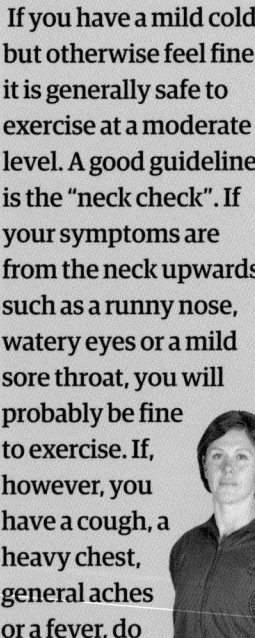

If you have a mild cold but otherwise feel fine, it is generally safe to exercise at a moderate level. A good guideline is the "neck check". If your symptoms are from the neck upwards, such as a runny nose, watery eyes or a mild sore throat, you will probably be fine to exercise. If, however, you have a cough, a heavy chest, general aches or a fever, do not exercise.

Personal safety

Exercising outdoors, particularly alone, requires a few simple precautions:

- Wear reflective or bright (high visibility) clothing so that you can be seen.
- Do not wear headphones when exercising where there is traffic or other hazards to your safety. You will not be alert and aware of your surroundings.
- Avoid exercising alone in unpopulated areas, or areas you are unfamiliar with.
- Carry a mobile phone and personal alarm with you.
- Let someone know where you are going and give them an estimate of how long you think you will be.
- Carry some form of identification with you in the event of an accident.

Exercise and health

Regular exercise is good for you, that's a given. But while some exercise is good, more is not necessarily better. Studies show that there is a limit beyond which exercise stops being beneficial to health and actually begins to compromise the immune system, so leaving you susceptible to coughs, colds and infections. That's why it is important not to overdo things (see Overtraining, below), to get sufficient sleep and to ensure you have plenty of rest built into your schedule.

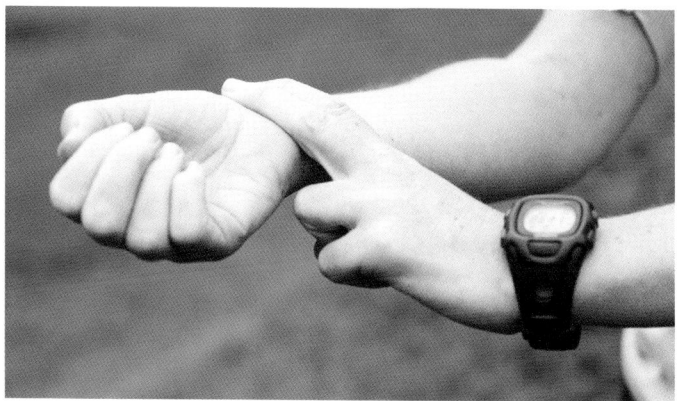

One sign that you are under the weather is an elevated resting heart rate. A reading of ten beats per minute or so higher than your usual rate indicates that you have not fully recovered from previous training or are about to come down with something. For the most accurate results, check your resting heart rate first thing in the morning. If it is higher than usual, this is a sign that you should get some rest instead of exercising. This is necessary to allow your body to recover.

Overtraining

If you are constantly tired, moody or irritable, if your limbs feel heavy, you suffer from frequent illnesses, have lost your appetite, are not sleeping well or are unable to perform to your expectations, you may have overtraining syndrome. This is accumulated fatigue, resulting from excessive training and inadequate recovery. Poor diet, particularly inadequate calorie intake, and insufficient carbohydrate and water consumption are other contributing factors. It may be worth a visit to your GP for blood tests to check there is no viral component.

The first step to take is to immediately decrease the volume and intensity of your training. If this doesn't help, you may need a period of complete rest from physical activity. Try easing off for a minimum of four weeks and see whether you regain your energy and enthusiasm for exercise. For women, if your periods have stopped or become irregular, see your doctor, as you may be losing valuable bone density and putting your health at risk.

Nutrition and performance

If you wish to get the best out of yourself, you need to make sure that you eat a healthy, balanced diet. That holds true whether you are an Army recruit, a busy mother or a stressed-out executive. But if you are also striving to improve fitness and get in great shape, it is doubly important that what you eat and drink successfully meets your body's needs.

The healthy balanced diet

If you get the balance between nutritional intake and exercise right you will achieve and maintain your ideal body weight, stay healthy, have lots of energy, improve your exercise performance, reduce your chances of being injured and recover more quickly from physical endeavours. Get it wrong, however, and no matter how hard you train, you simply will not achieve what you are capable of.

In simple terms, a healthy balanced diet means the right type of food and drink, consumed in the right quantities. We all need certain nutrients in order to be healthy. But while the basic principles remain the same, there are a few differences between the dietary needs of someone who is physically active on a regular basis and those of the average couch potato. Generally, a physically active person needs:

- A higher total calorie intake, to meet increased energy expenditure.
- A lot more carbohydrate, the body's preferred fuel source for physical activity.
- A little more protein, to repair the damage done by training.
- A higher fluid intake, to offset the losses caused by sweating.
- Lower fat consumption, to allow for greater carbohydrate intake and help maintain appropriate body weight for maximum performance.

Carbohydrate

For an active lifestyle, the most important nutrient is carbohydrate, so this should be present on your plate at every meal and snack. In fact, carbohydrate-rich foods should make up more than half your total daily calorie intake.

The reason carbohydrate is so important in your diet is that it is the main source of fuel for physical activity - the body converts it into glucose, which is transported to the working muscles by the blood.

Carbohydrate is stored in the muscles as a substance called glycogen, and because the body has a limited capacity for storage, supplies need to be constantly replenished.

Carbohydrate-rich foods include sugary foods like jam, sweets and fruit juices as well as starchy foods like potatoes, rice, grains, pasta and bread. The sugary foods (and highly-

What to put in your shopping trolley

CARBOHYDRATE

- Wholegrain pasta
- Porridge oats
- Sweet potato
- Beans
- Noodles
- Brown rice
- Basmati rice

- New potatoes
- Rye bread
- Muesli
- Malt loaf
- Oatcakes
- Dried apricots
- Dried figs

refined starches, such as white bread or rice and sugary breakfast cereals) flood the blood with glucose very rapidly, while more "complex" carbohydrates, like porridge oats, brown rice and wholegrain bread, release their sugar more slowly.

The speed at which a food releases its sugar into the bloodstream is measured by what is known as the glycaemic index (GI). Low-GI carbohydrates release energy slowly, while high-GI choices increase blood glucose very quickly, which can lead to an energy rush, followed by a low. Generally speaking, it is healthier to opt for low-GI carbohydrates most of the time. Too many high-GI carbs can play havoc with insulin levels and excessive consumption has been linked to the onset of Type 2 diabetes.

That said, high-GI foods can be useful for physical activity. Research from the University of Sydney has found that athletes eating high-GI foods do not get the same "spike" in insulin levels that sedentary people experience. There's no need to outlaw high-GI foods altogether, therefore, but you should consume them less

PTI Tip

Choose wholegrain breakfast cereals such as Weetabix, Shredded Wheat or porridge oats rather than sugar-coated varieties such as Coco Pops and Frosties.

frequently than their healthier low-GI siblings.

As far as how much carbohydrate you need is concerned, a general rule of thumb is to aim for 60% of your overall calorie intake, a slightly higher level than that recommended for someone who is sedentary. The American College of Sports Medicine bases its recommended intake on body weight and training level, suggesting a range from 6-10g of carbohydrate per kg of body weight.

Protein

Protein forms our muscles and is a vital nutrient in body repair and growth. If you are very active (regularly exercising a few times a week), you need slightly more protein than the recommended average (1.2-1.4g of protein per kg of body weight per day compared to 0.75g for a sedentary person). However, most of us already eat more protein than we need, so it is unlikely that you will need to make a special effort to consume more. And increasing your protein consumption beyond the recommended levels will not necessarily make you any stronger. In fact, there is no scientific evidence to support the idea.

What *is* important is to choose good-quality sources of protein-rich foods – ideally those that do not come complete with high levels of saturated fat. Good choices include lean red meat, fish (particularly oily fish, for its healthy omega 3 content), poultry, eggs and low-fat dairy products (which are a great source of calcium). Non-animal sources of protein, such as beans and pulses, nuts, seeds, tofu and soya are also good options.

Fat

Fat is essential in the human diet but, in general, most of us consume more than we need, leading to excess body fat and to an increased risk of many chronic diseases. While carbohydrate and protein contain around 4 calories per gram, fat contains 9 calories per gram, making it a very energy-dense nutrient that is easy to overconsume.

One military study found that Army Phase 1 recruits were consuming 42% of their overall calories from fat, which is 7% higher than the government guideline of a maximum of 35%. If you are active and keen to maximise your performance gains through healthy eating, you need to aim for lower fat levels, in order to accommodate the higher level of carbohydrate. The American College of Sports Medicine's recommendation of 25% of total calories from fat for physically active individuals is a sensible target. You will also need to reduce your fat intake if you are trying to lose body weight. Fat is present in our diet not just in its visible form, such as in butter, oil or fatty meats, but also in its hidden form – in processed foods, fast food and takeaways.

You can lower your fat intake by choosing leaner meats, removing the fat and skin from meat, swapping full-fat products for low-fat alternatives and choosing skimmed or semi-skimmed milk instead of full fat. Reduce the number of high-fat snacks you eat, such as crisps, pasties and chips.

As well as watching how much fat we eat, we should take care to eat healthier *types* of fat. For example, the saturated fat found in burgers, creamy sauces and

What to put in your shopping trolley

PROTEIN

- Extra lean minced beef
- Turkey or chicken breasts
- Eggs
- Skimmed or semi-skimmed milk
- Low-fat yoghurt
- Sunflower and pumpkin seeds
- Salmon fillets
- Mackerel or sardines tinned in spring water
- Red kidney beans
- Lentils

What to put in your shopping trolley

FAT

- Olive oil
- Rapeseed or soya oil
- Low-fat dairy products
- avocados
- Oily fish
- Nuts and seeds
- Peanut butter

meat pies is unhealthy for the heart, while unsaturated fat (including the omega 3 fatty acids found in oily fish) and the monounsaturated fats derived from vegetable sources such as avocados and olive oil are healthier.

Vitamins, minerals and fibre

Carbohydrate, fat and protein are the key nutrients in our diet. But these must be supported by sufficient intake of vitamins and minerals, and fibre - a component of food that bulks it out, aiding digestion. Some foods, such as breakfast cereals and fruit juices, are "fortified" with vitamins and minerals, but it is best to get most of your daily intake from natural sources. Fruit and vegetables are a rich source of fibre, vitamins and minerals as well as antioxidants, which help to repair the damage done by training.

Aim for a wide range of produce, rather than sticking to apples and bananas, in order to get the best range of vitamins and minerals possible. Green leafy vegetables like spinach and kale are good sources of iron, while strawberries, oranges and kiwis are high in vitamin C, for example.

You will have heard the "five a day" message - the government's advice that we eat at least five portions of fruit and vegetables each day. Well, it is easier than you think. One of those five portions can be a juice and one can be dried fruit. Throw in a banana, a salad with lunch and a helping or two of vegetables with dinner and you've exceeded the target. Also bear in mind that fruit and vegetables can be fresh, frozen or canned. So think canned sweetcorn kernels, frozen peas and tinned pineapple as well as fresh produce.

The non-nutrients

A healthy diet is as much about what you *do not* eat as what you do eat.

Consuming too much salt can have a detrimental effect on your health, particularly on your blood pressure. So if your blood pressure is high or borderline, avoid excessive salt intake. The easiest way to reduce your salt intake is to stop adding it to your food. Many foods are already full of

DID YOU KNOW?

Potatoes, despite being a vegetable, do not count towards your five-a-day target.

PTI Tip

If a product is labelled "low fat" this does not mean you can eat endless quantities of it. Use the same amount of low-fat spread or dip as you would a higher-fat version.

sodium (from which salt is formed). Cutting down on salty snacks like crisps and salted nuts and reducing your intake of highly processed foods will also help. The UK government advises eating no more than 6 grams of salt a day (2.4g of sodium) – about one level teaspoon.

Many soldiers like the odd drink when they are off duty but are aware that excessive alcohol intake will have an effect on their physical performance and so drink in moderation. Alcohol affects you not only at the time of drinking (interfering with reaction speed and coordination) but it also contributes to dehydration and hampers recovery, so

even a day or so after you've drunk too much, your body will still be feeling the effects. Alcohol is also very high in calories, containing 7 calories per gram. Men should not consume more than 21 units of alcohol per week; women should not exceed 14 units. One unit is equal to half a pint of beer or a small glass of wine (125ml/4.5fl oz).

Energy balance explained

Now that you have a clearer idea of what you should be eating, what about quantity? Your own specific energy requirements are unique to you. The government's guidelines for the general population are a useful reference point – they recommend a daily intake of 2,550 calories for men and 1,940 for women. That is fine for the average sedentary person, but it is unlikely to be sufficient to fuel regular physical activity. To give you an idea, our statistics show that a UK Phase 1 male Army recruit burns approximately 3,570 calories per day while a female uses 2,960 calories. In general, the

DID YOU KNOW?

You can calculate the amount of salt in a food by multiplying the value given for sodium on the food's label by 2.5. For example, if sodium is listed as 0.2g per serving, the actual salt content is 0.2x2.5=0.5g

PTI Tip

When it comes to fruit and veg, the more colourful the better, in terms of vitamins, minerals and phytochemicals. Try red peppers, peaches, sweet potatoes and pink grapefruit to begin with.

bigger you are, the more calories you burn per day. Women burn fewer calories than men, while older and less fit people burn fewer calories than younger, fitter individuals.

Estimating your energy needs

If you have a healthy body weight, and are maintaining that weight, you are eating the right number of calories and achieving "energy balance", where energy intake (from the food and drink you consume) is equal to energy output (the energy you expend during the day). If you are losing or gaining weight, then you are in a "negative" or "positive" energy balance situation.

Here's a way of estimating your individual energy requirement. This formula is based on your "basal metabolic rate" (BMR), which is the amount of energy required by your body simply to "tick over", and your "physical activity level" (PAL), a score based on how active you are in daily life.

Calculate your BMR using the table below and write it in the box at the bottom of the page:

age	male	female
10-17	BMR = (17.7 x BW) + 657	BMR = (13.4 x BW) + 692
18-29	BMR = (15.1 x BW) + 692	BMR = (14.8 x BW) + 487
30-59	BMR = (11.5 x BW) + 873	BMR = (8.3 x BW) + 846
BMR = basal metabolic rate	BW = body weight in kg (1kg = 2.2lbs)	

Now check your PAL score using the table below and write it in the box at the bottom of the page:

activity level	male and female
non-active	1.4
moderately active	1.5
very active	1.6
PAL= physical activity level	

To get your estimated daily energy requirement multiply your BMR score by your PAL score.

Example: A moderately active 30-year-old male with a body weight of 70kg has a BMR of 1,678 and a PAL score of 1.5. Therefore his estimated energy requirement is 1,678 (BMR) x 1.5 (PAL) = 2,517 calories.

Your BMR =	Your PAL =
(BMR) x (PAL) = your daily energy requirement (in calories)	
=	

What's in a good drink?

A good sports drink contains carbohydrate in the form of different sugars (such as glucose, fructose and sucrose) along with electrolyte salts (which are lost from the body through sweat) such as sodium and potassium. An "isotonic" formula, which contains 6-8g of carbohydrate per 100ml, is most easily absorbed. A higher concentration than this will mean slower uptake of the fluid and is not ideal during exercise. It is, however, fine as a post-training drink.

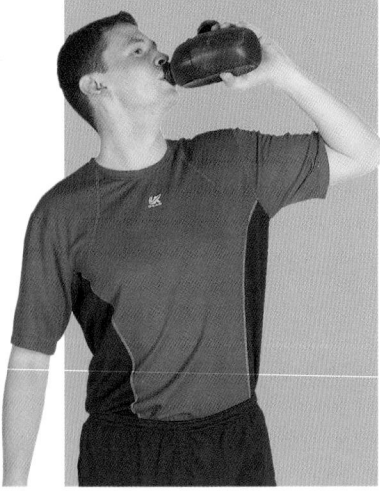

Losing weight

We've talked about ensuring you have sufficient calorie intake for increased activity, but what if you *need* to lose weight? (You can get a reasonable guideline by filling in the BMI chart on p.113.)

Here, the goal is twofold: to reduce your energy intake a little, and increase your energy output a little. It is a more effective strategy to do both of these in moderation rather than to attempt to cut your calorie intake in half or exercise to extremes. Research shows that drastic dietary changes result only in temporary weight loss. For sustained weight loss, it is best to make small changes that you can continue with in the longer term. Naturally, given the importance of carbohydrate for a physically active lifestyle, the Army does not recommend low-carbohydrate diets as a weight-loss method.

Fluid intake

Water is essential to human life – it is present in all the body's cells and accounts for approximately 66% of our total body weight. Maintaining correct fluid levels is important at all times, but especially so during exercise, because sweating causes the body to lose more water. If you do not drink as much as you need to, you will become dehydrated and this will have a detrimental effect on your mental and physical performance (and can be extremely dangerous).

But how do you know how much water you need? It depends on many factors: individual differences, the conditions in which you are exercising, what you are wearing and the type, intensity and length of the exercise you are engaged in. According to the American College of Sports Medicine's 2007 guidelines, there is no set figure, because sweat rates, and the electrolyte content of that sweat, varies too widely from person to person. In other words, you need to establish your own

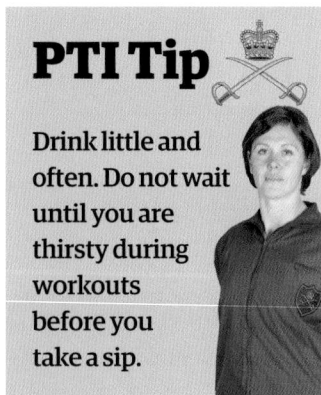

PTI Tip

Drink little and often. Do not wait until you are thirsty during workouts before you take a sip.

hydration needs. Weighing yourself before and after exercise (your weight loss in grams is equal to your water loss in ml) will help. You can also use the urine test, below.

The urine test

Check your urine: its colour is a good indicator of your hydration level. Small volumes of dark, strong-smelling urine indicate dehydration while large volumes of light-coloured urine are a sign that you are well hydrated.

Avoiding dehydration

- Drink sports drinks, which contain electrolytes and carbohydrates as well as water. This is particularly important during longer exercise sessions (60 minutes or more).
- Carry fluid with you during workouts.
- Pay attention to what and how much you're drinking during the day to ensure you are well hydrated when you start exercise.

Fuelling physical performance

Soldiers with physically demanding jobs need to pay as much attention to their diet as athletes. Good nutrition

Nutrition and injury prevention

A healthy balanced diet may even help you stay injury free and recover better from injuries.

Evidence suggests that good nutrition can delay the onset of muscle fatigue. When muscles get tired, they are less efficient at absorbing the forces generated by impact, putting the bones and joints under greater stress. On a more long-term basis, good nutrition – particularly calcium intake and sufficient calorie intake – is important in preventing stress fractures, which are a particular problem in female military recruits.

alone will not make a good athlete, but it will make a good athlete better.

Good nutrition for the physically active differs slightly from that for the less or non-active, mainly because of the increased overall energy and fluid requirement and the need for a higher intake of carbohydrate. Also, high-GI carbohydrates (p. 157) can be a positive contribution to physical training. Firstly, they ensure that glucose is delivered to the blood quickly so it can be used instantly. Secondly, they can be consumed "on the run" in the form of sport drinks or energy gels, so you don't run out of energy during a long workout. It has been shown that for exercise lasting 60 minutes or

more, ingesting carbohydrate aids performance more than does water alone.

Finally, high-GI carbs help to facilitate the post-exercise recovery process. Research suggests that during the couple of hours after exercise, carbohydrates consumed will be laid down as glycogen more efficiently than at other times. Aim for 1g of carbohydrate per kg of your body weight in this post-workout snack, and ensure that your subsequent meals are rich in good-quality carbohydrates. Research has shown that if you consume protein with your carbohydrate snack you maximise absorption. The protein also assists with muscle repair and recovery.

Clothing, footwear and equipment

You do not need lots of special clothing or equipment to get fit with the Army - the simplicity of the programmes is part of their appeal. But you do need the right footwear. While soldiers may wear heavy-duty boots for marching, running shoes are always used for running to help reduce the risk of injury. You, too, should ensure that your footwear is specific to the activity you are performing because a shoe's structure and support will differ, depending on the purpose for which it is designed.

Running shoes

Running involves high-impact, repetitive landings, so it is particularly important that you have a good-quality pair of trainers for your workouts. So what should you look for in a pair of running shoes? The main factors are comfort, cushioning, stability, responsiveness and durability. There is no single brand or model of running shoe that is right for everyone. We all have different foot shapes, different "gait" patterns (the way we walk or run) and other individual differences (for example, body weight, the terrain we will be covering, the number of miles and the pace at which we move). Different shoes are geared towards these needs. For example, some are highly cushioned, while others are stiffer and more stable.

The "wet footprint" test (p.166) will help give you an idea of your foot type and shape. It is best to buy your running shoes from a specialist retailer to ensure you get the best advice and choice. And bear in mind you may have to go up or down a shoe size to get the right fit.

Finally, ensure that your running shoes are in good condition - worn-out or damaged trainers will not provide the essential support and protection you need. In general, running shoes will last for 300-500 miles (500-800kms).

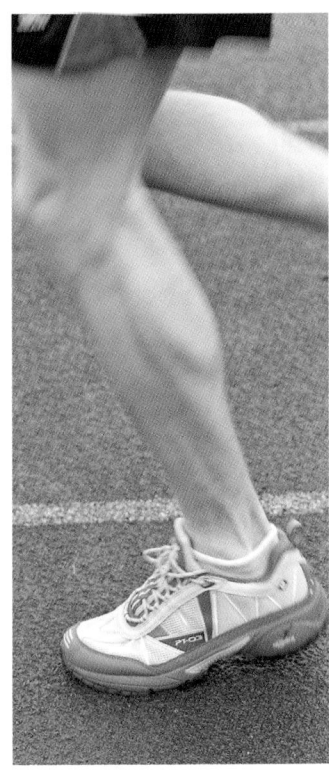

The shoe in detail

OUTSOLE: the rubber outer layer that sits under the shoe. "Lugs" on its surface help to enhance traction and grip.

INSOLE: a removable layer inside, primarily for comfort.

HEEL COUNTER: the area that cups the heel. This should not dig into the Achilles tendon.

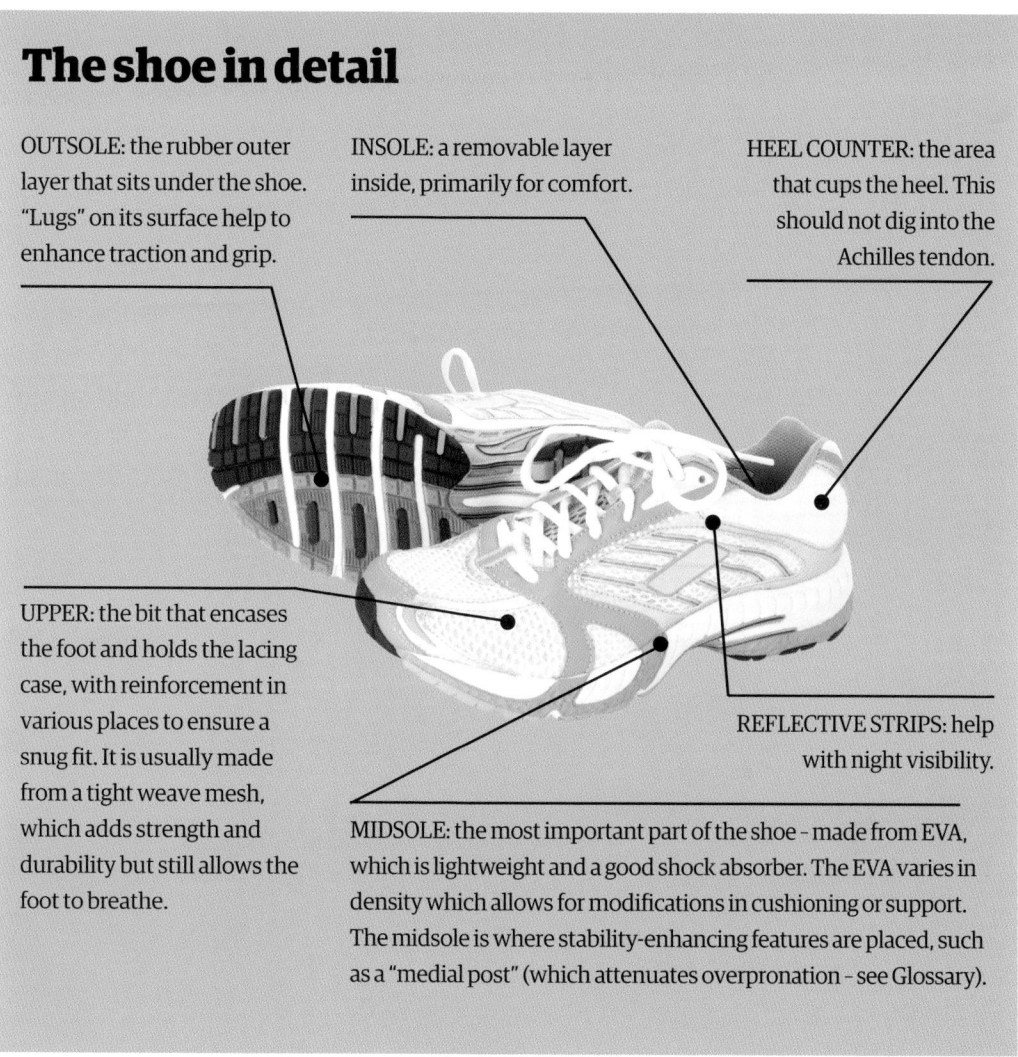

UPPER: the bit that encases the foot and holds the lacing case, with reinforcement in various places to ensure a snug fit. It is usually made from a tight weave mesh, which adds strength and durability but still allows the foot to breathe.

REFLECTIVE STRIPS: help with night visibility.

MIDSOLE: the most important part of the shoe - made from EVA, which is lightweight and a good shock absorber. The EVA varies in density which allows for modifications in cushioning or support. The midsole is where stability-enhancing features are placed, such as a "medial post" (which attenuates overpronation - see Glossary).

Footwear for other sports

Running shoes are suitable for walking on even ground if you do not have walking shoes or boots because both walking and running are linear activities. However, they are not ideal for multi-directional activities, such as tennis or circuit training. If you are moving laterally, a running shoe does not provide sufficient stability to prevent you turning on your ankle. In addition, the lack of forefoot cushioning does not provide much shock absorption for high-impact landings. A pair of good-quality cross-trainers or sport-specific shoes (for example, tennis shoes or basketball boots) is the best choice if you are going to do a lot of non-linear activities.

The wet footprint test

The wet footprint test gives you hints about your foot type and gait pattern, by providing an imprint of your foot. Dunk your feet in water and then take a few steps across a patch of concrete (or anywhere that will leave a visible imprint.) Then compare what you see with the shapes below. This test will give you an idea of what type of shoe to ask for in a sports shop.

Normal (medium) arch

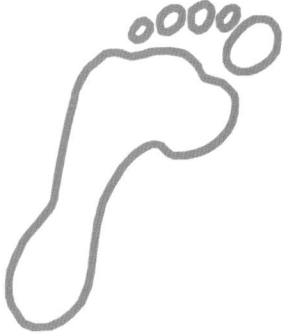

Normal feet, with a normal arch, will display the forefoot and heel connected by a broad band. A normal foot lands on the outside of the heel and rolls inwards slightly to absorb shock (this is called "pronation"). An appropriate shoe is one which allows this to take place without over-controlling it.

Best shoes: Neutral shoes, stability shoes with moderate control.

Flat (low) arch

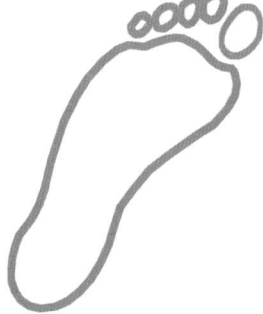

If you can see almost your entire footprint, you have a flat foot with a low arch, which is indicative of overpronation (meaning your foot rolls in too quickly or too much on foot strike). Shoes that are designed to attenuate this help reduce the risk of injuries and provide support and stability.

Best shoes: Stability shoes with medial support, motion control shoes.

High arch

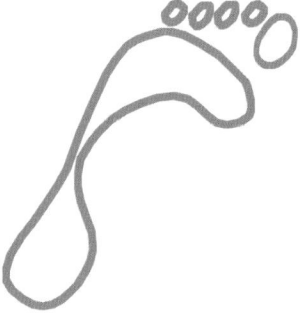

A narrow band - or no band at all - linking the ball of the foot to the heel demonstrates a high-arched foot. This type of foot generally does not pronate enough, which reduces its efficiency as a shock absorber. This foot type needs a shoe that provides good cushioning. Avoid stability shoes or shoes with medial support as these will exacerbate the problem.

Best shoes: Cushioned shoes with plenty of flexibility.

What to wear

Clothing for physical training should be comfortable and non-restrictive. Technical fabrics have the advantage of being breathable and sweat-wicking, so you stay cool and dry in them. But a cotton t-shirt will also do just fine. In cooler climes, dress in thin layers so that you can remove one as you warm up. Stay away from thick, heavy fabrics that will get drenched in sweat and end up chafing.

Sports sunglasses will protect your eyes from UV rays, grit and pollution, and prevent eye fatigue. A cap or visor will keep the sun off. In cold weather, gloves and a hat help you retain body heat.

Heart-rate monitors, GPSs and other gadgets

The only gadget you really need for the Army Fitness Programmes is a watch, so that you can keep tabs on your timing (particularly during interval and circuit training). But technology can be very motivating, and one of the best pieces of equipment you can invest in is a heart-rate monitor. This device, which consists of a chest strap and a watch to which your heart rate is transmitted, enables you to check how hard you are working, and ensures you are neither taking it too easy nor overdoing it. Basic models simply monitor and record your heart rate during an exercise session while more complex ones can determine your "training zones", record calorie expenditure and fat utilisation and, when coupled with a foot pod, measure your pace and distance. Another option for tracking speed and distance - as well as your exact route and location - is a global positioning system (GPS) monitor. Top-of-the-range options combine a heart-rate monitor and GPS device so that you can get data on everything you could possibly want to know about your training.

Another gizmo worth considering is a pedometer. This simple device clips on to your waistband or belt and counts your strides (by registering the movement of your hips). If you take a measurement of your average stride length, a pedometer can estimate how much ground you've covered. They are less accurate on hilly terrain as running up or down hills alters stride length.

Drinking vessels

It is important to stay hydrated when you are training (read more on page 162), so take fluid with you on longer sessions, or when it is hot. A simple drink bottle is fine if you are exercising in a single place, but if you are on the move, a bottle with a moulded grip and sports cap is useful. If you wish to keep your hands free, a hydration pack (a small rucksack with an internal bladder) is a great idea. A long straw reaches round from the pack to your mouth, so you do not need to stop running (or walking) to take a drink.

Exercise equipment

The exercise programmes in this book do not require access to a gym, and use only minimal equipment. Even if you do not have the equipment used here, it is often easy to improvise, using common household items.

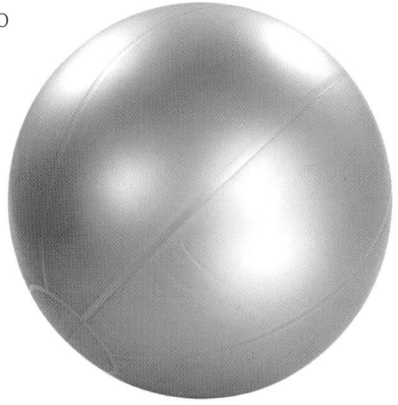

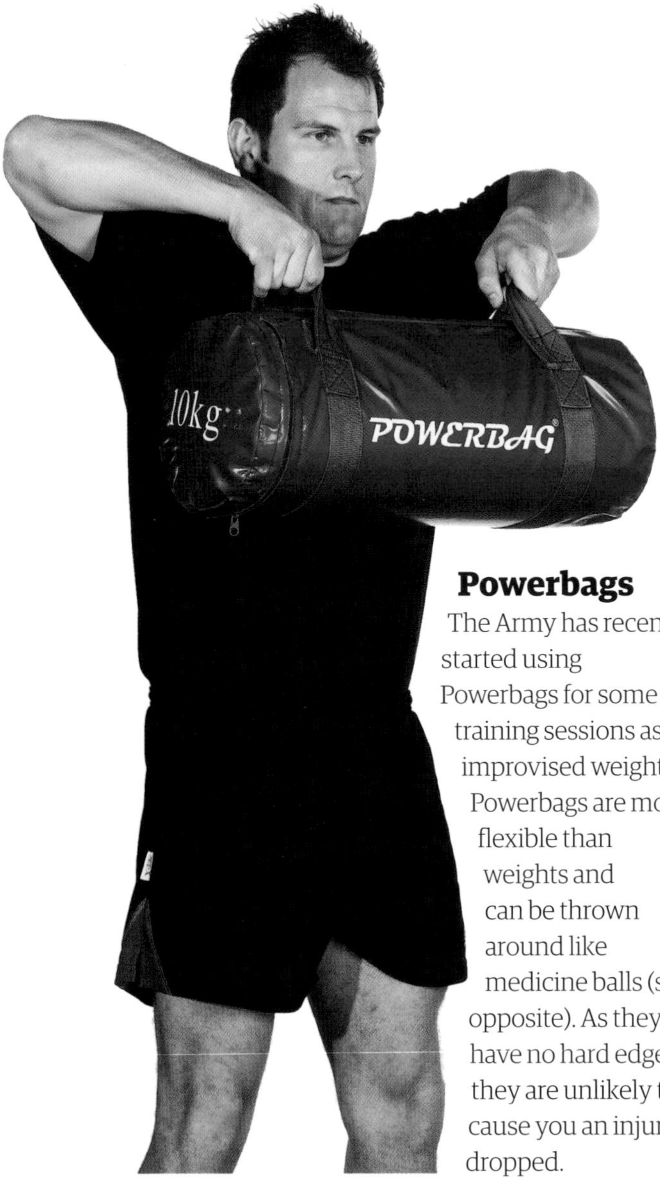

Swiss balls

A Swiss ball makes a good exercise tool (see the exercises on pages 73-75). It creates an unstable surface on which to exercise, so you are forced to use the stabilising muscles more to help you maintain your position. It is important to get the right size Swiss ball for your height. Use the guidelines below to help you choose. When you sit on the ball your hips should be slightly higher than your knees.

Powerbags

The Army has recently started using Powerbags for some training sessions as improvised weights. Powerbags are more flexible than weights and can be thrown around like medicine balls (see opposite). As they have no hard edges, they are unlikely to cause you an injury if dropped.

Your height	Swiss ball size
5ft–5ft 5in (1.52m–1.65m)	55cm (1ft 9in) ball
5ft 6in–6ft 1in (1.68m–1.85m)	65cm (2ft 1in) ball
6ft 2in–6ft 8in (1.88m–2.03m)	75cm (2ft 5in) ball

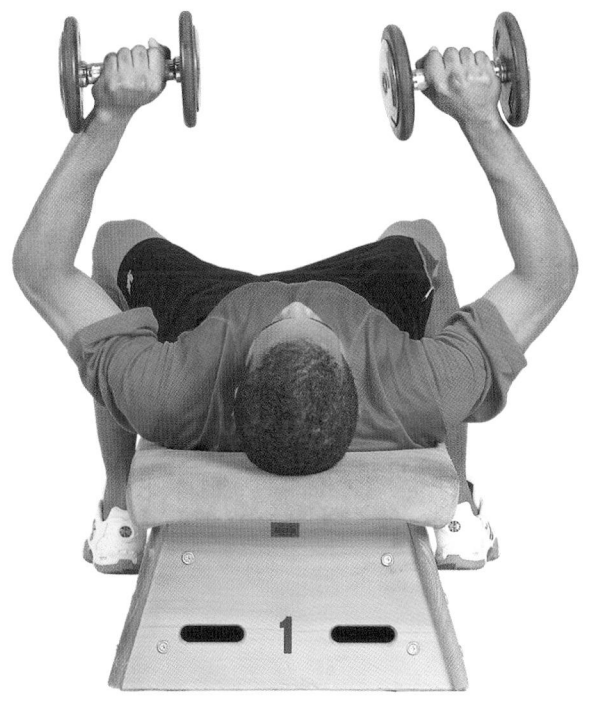

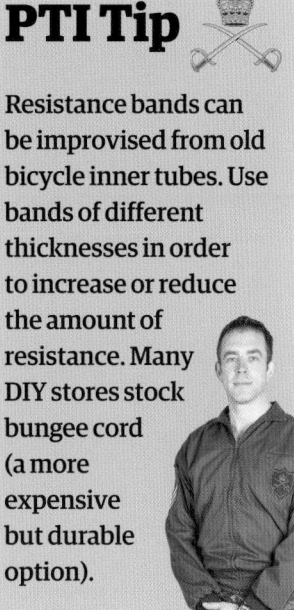
Medicine balls

This classic piece of exercise equipment has recently made a comeback and is commonly found in gyms and other training environments. Medicine balls are about the size of a football, and of varying weights. They enable you to perform strength and power exercises, such as the Prone Hamstring Curl (p.70).

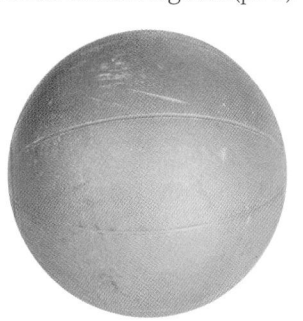

Steps

A step is a versatile piece of fitness equipment. You can use it as a platform to step up and down from, or set it up as a makeshift weights bench, either flat or set on an incline. Adjustable "risers" allow you to alter the height of the step, too.

Elastic resistance

Resistance bands or tubes are a great way of performing strength training if you do not have weights or access to a gym. Different levels of resistance are available. A useful accompanying gadget is a "door attachment", which

you thread around the tube to enable you to secure the band to the top of a doorframe and perform overhead exercises (for example, see the Lat Pull-Down page 67).

Staying motivated

Fitting regular physical activity into a busy life is always a challenge. But having clear goals about what you wish to achieve, and knowing the steps you need to take in order to achieve them, helps you stay focused and motivated. That is why goal-setting is such an important process.

Setting SMARTER goals

It is important to have short, medium and long-term goals. For example, you may eventually want to run a full marathon, but in the meantime you could start by setting your sights on a half marathon – with a short-term goal to increase your running distance by 1-2 miles per week. Without these more immediate goals, long-term goals can feel distant and remote - as if you will never get there. Think of it as laying stepping stones along the path to your destination.

Once you have formulated your goals, check that they comply with the SMARTER acronym:

S - Goals must be **Specific**.
M - Training targets should be **Measurable**.
A - Goals should be **Agreed**, if relevant, with a coach, personal trainer or a workout companion.

R - Goals must be **Realistic** and achievable.
T - Training targets should be **Time-framed**, counting back from specific dates, where possible (for example, a particular race).
E - Goals should be **Exciting**, to keep you motivated.
R - Goals should be **Recorded**. Writing things down makes them feel more real than when they are simply in your head. Recorded goals also mean that it is easier to make adjustments to the programme, where necessary. Example: "I want to better my 2.4-km run time by at least 30 seconds by the end of the 12-week programme that I've just started."

Checking off your goals against the SMARTER principles will increase your chances of reaching them successfully by ruling out unrealistic aims, turning

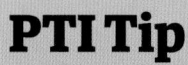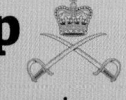

PTI Tip

The words you use in stating your goal are important. For example, compare "I must stop eating so much junk" to "I will make healthier eating choices". Negative words and phrases like "give up" and "ought to" or "should" are much less powerful than positive statements like "I will" and "I want".

vague ideas into concrete ones and by committing them to paper.

But the goal-setting process does not end the

moment you begin training. It is important to regularly revisit and reassess your goals as you monitor your progress. A training journal, in which you record the details of what you have achieved in each session, is a very helpful way of keeping track. A written record of your achievements (or, as the case may be, your lack of achievements) serves as a strong motivator. It is also helpful to look back and see which sessions worked best for you, so you can continue to incorporate them in future training plans.

Get organised

Goal-setting is one way of increasing your chances of success. But you will also make training easier if you are organised. For example, you should have all the equipment and clothing you need for your fitness programme at hand so you do not have to waste time looking for it. Schedule your training into your diary, so that you do not run out of time and end up being unable to fit a workout in. Book courts, classes and sessions in advance, rather than leaving it to the last minute and finding there's no

space. Even with the best intentions, exercise can fall off the agenda in a hectic, disorganised routine.

You may find that incorporating exercise into your usual routine is a good way of getting it done with minimal upheaval. For example, running or cycling to work or fitting in sessions during your lunch break.

Four ways to stay on track

■ Finding a workout companion can really help you stay motivated. You are much more likely to turn up for a training session if

you have arranged to meet someone than if you have planned to do it alone. You may choose to exercise with a friend or partner. But proceed with caution if the person you choose has a fitness level or build that is very different from yours – take care not to overdo it, or push them too far beyond their comfort zone.

■ If you cannot manage your usual workout, make sure you do at least 10 minutes. At the end of that period, see how you feel. More often than not, you will be ready to carry on, but if you do not feel up to it,

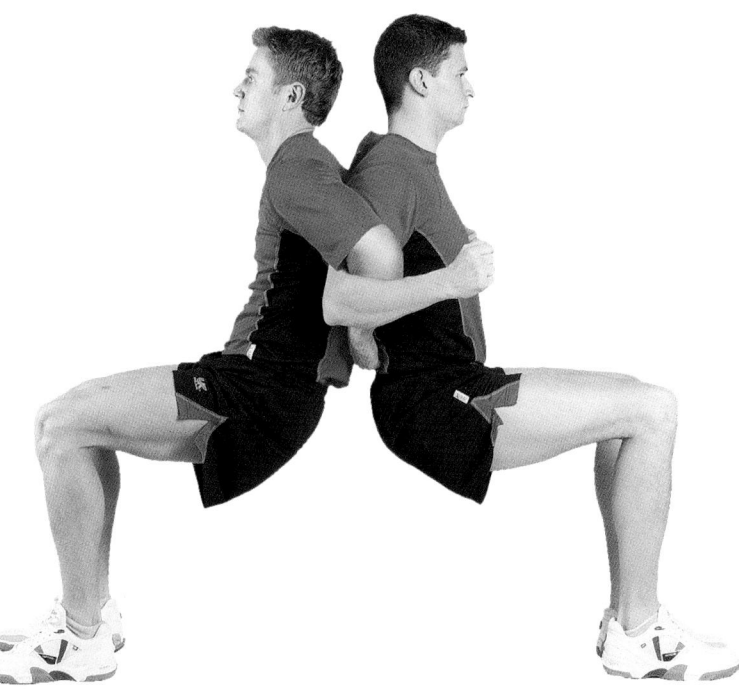

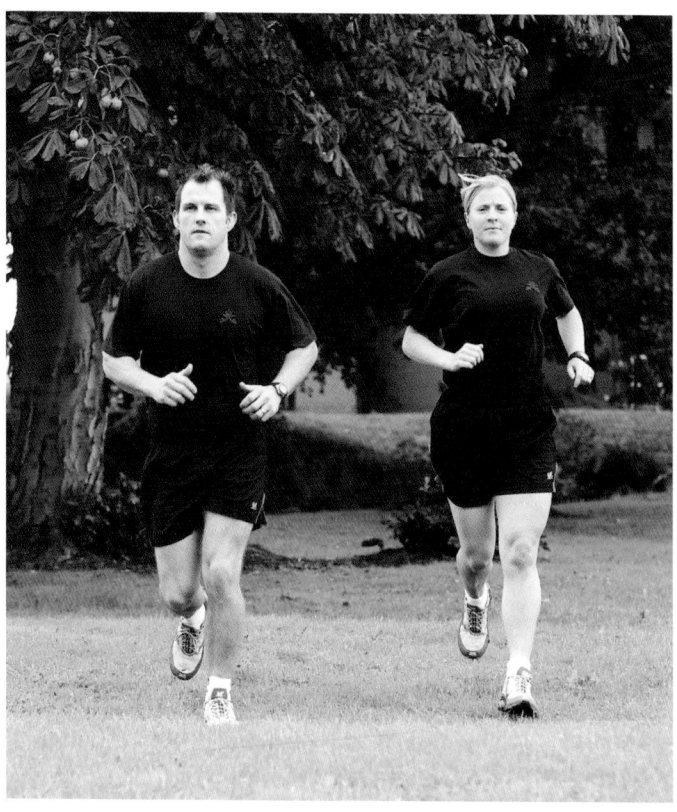

Good timing

Does the time of day at which you exercise matter? Experts stress that while there is some evidence that the body is more geared up for exercise at some periods of the day than at others, the most important thing is that you do it at all.

The notion that you should do what feels right for you was backed up by a study published in the journal *Medicine and Science in Sports and Exercise*. The study found that people who always trained either in the morning or evening and were then asked to perform a high-intensity workout to exhaustion did better if they performed the workout at their usual exercise time. But just for the record, research suggests that the body is most primed for activity between 4 and 7pm.

remember that it is OK to skip the odd session. If, however, you regularly feel unable to do your workouts, you should try to determine why. Perhaps your diet isn't providing sufficient energy to fuel your efforts? Or perhaps you are pushing yourself too hard with a programme that is beyond your current abilities? Set yourself some new, achievable targets.

- Reward yourself for sticking to your regime. Ideally with something connected to fitness rather than with a few beers and a pizza. Try a sports massage or buy some new exercise clothing or equipment each time you complete one of the programmes.

- Gadgets can help you stay motivated. Heart-rate monitors and exercise-specific GPS devices will often be accompanied by a software-based training diary which you can use to record progress and set goals.

So get going!

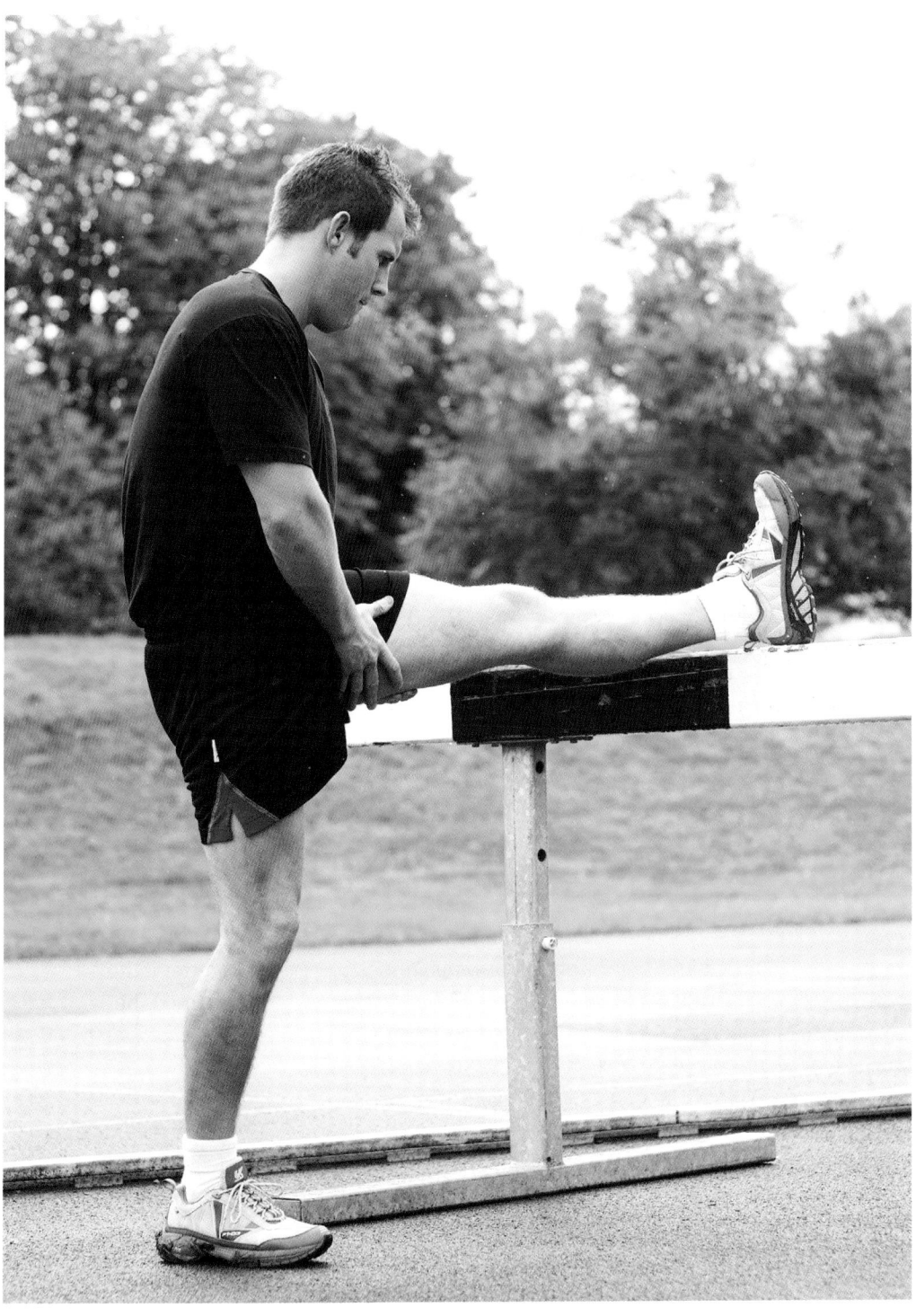

Glossary

Acute injury An injury that has occurred recently

Adaptation The process by which the body adapts to a more challenging exercise load

Aerobic fitness/endurance The ability to carry out prolonged physical activity and resist fatigue. Dependent on the body's efficiency in taking in and utilising oxygen

Anaerobic exercise Exercise of high intensity but short duration which does not rely on oxygen

Antioxidant A substance that prevents or attenuates oxidation, a process that is linked to the production of harmful free radicals

Basal metabolic rate The rate of metabolism at complete rest

Body mass index (BMI) A calculation to estimate body composition

Cadence The rate of foot strike or pedal revolutions per minute

Cardiorespiratory Referring to the heart and lungs

Cardiovascular Referring to the heart, blood and blood vessels

Chronic injury An injury that develops over time

Compound exercise An exercise that uses multiple muscle groups and joints

Core stability Appropriate strength and function of the stabilising muscles in the trunk area of the body

Cross training Maintaining or improving performance by engaging in activities other than your main sport or activity

Dehydration A detrimental loss of fluid from the body

Delayed Onset Muscle Soreness (DOMS) Muscle soreness that develops in the 24-48 hours post exercise

Dynamic In motion

Electrolytes Mineral salts (mainly sodium and potassium) lost through sweat

Energy expenditure The amount of energy used in a given task, measured in calories

Fartlek A running training session, where speed and terrain are varied at will to place the aerobic and anaerobic systems under stress

Free radical An atom with at least one unpaired electron, that is either produced in the body or introduced from an outside source (e.g., tobacco smoke or pollutants) and can damage cells, proteins and DNA by altering their chemical structure

Glycaemic index (GI) A classification of the effect that a carbohydrate food has on blood sugar levels

Hypertension High blood pressure

Interval training High-intensity bouts of exercise separated by recovery periods

Isolated exercise An exercise that focuses on only one muscle group or joint

Isotonic A fluid with the same concentration as the body's fluids, allowing for faster absorption

Lactate threshold The point at which lactic acid (a by-product of metabolism)